Interpersonal Psychotherapy

EDITED BY
John C. Markowitz, M.D.

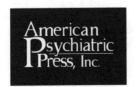

WASHINGTON, DC
LONDON, ENGLAND

Copyright © 1998 American Psychiatric Press, Inc.
First Edition   01   00   99   98   4   3   2
ALL RIGHTS RESERVED
Manufactured in the United States of America on acid-free paper

American Psychiatric Press, Inc.
1400 K Street, N.W.
Washington, DC   20005
www.appi.org

Library of Congress Cataloging-in-Publication Data

Interpersonal psychotherapy / edited by John C. Markowitz.
        p.   cm. — (Review of psychiatry series, ISSN 1041-5882)
    Includes bibliographical references and index.
    ISBN 0-88048-836-0 (paperbound : alk paper)
    1. Interpersonal psychotherapy. I. Markowitz, John C., 1954– II. Series.
    [DNLM: 1. Psychotherapy—methods. 2. Professional-Patient Relations.
    3. Depressive Disorder—therapy. WM 420 I62 1998]
    RC489.I55I58   1998
    616.89'14—dc21
    DNLM/DLC
    for Library of Congress   98-10859
                                                                                    CIP

British Library Cataloguing in Publication Data
A CIP record is available from the British Library.

Contents

Contributors

Christopher G. Fairburn, D.M., F.R.C.Psych.
Wellcome Principal Research Fellow and Professor of
Psychiatry, Department of Psychiatry, University of Oxford,
Oxford, England

Ellen Frank, Ph.D. Professor of Psychiatry and
Psychology, Department of Psychiatry, University of Pittsburgh
Medical Center, Western Psychiatric Institute and Clinic,
Pittsburgh, Pennsylvania

John C. Markowitz, M.D. Associate Professor of Clinical
Psychiatry and Director, Psychotherapy Clinic, Cornell
University Medical College, New York, New York

Donna Moreau, M.D. Research Scientist, New York State
Psychiatric Institute; Associate Clinical Professor of Child
Psychiatry in Psychiatry, Columbia University College of
Physicians and Surgeons; and Director, Children's Anxiety and
Depression Clinic, Presbyterian Hospital, New York, New York

Laura Mufson, Ph.D. Research Scientist, New York State
Psychiatric Institute; Assistant Professor of Clinical Psychology
in Psychiatry, Columbia University College of Physicians and
Surgeons; and Director of Training in Child Psychiatry

John M. Oldham, M.D. Director, New York State
Psychiatric Institute; and Professor and Vice Chairman,
Department of Psychiatry, Columbia University College of
Physicians and Surgeons, New York, New York

Michelle B. Riba, M.D. Clinical Associate Professor of
Psychiatry and Associate Chair for Education and Academic
Affairs, Department of Psychiatry, University of Michigan
Health System, Ann Arbor, Michigan

Cynthia Spanier, Ph.D.   Post-Doctoral Fellow, Department of Psychiatry, University of Pittsburgh Medical Center, Western Psychiatric Institute and Clinic, Pittsburgh, Pennsylvania

Holly A. Swartz, M.D.   Assistant Professor of Psychiatry, Department of Psychiatry, University of Pittsburgh Medical Center, Western Psychiatric Institute and Clinic, Pittsburgh, Pennsylvania

Myrna M. Weissman, Ph.D.   Professor of Epidemiology in Psychiatry, Columbia University College of Physicians and Surgeons; and Chief, Division of Clinical and Genetic Epidemiology, New York State Psychiatric Institute, New York, New York

Introduction to the Review of Psychiatry Series

John M. Oldham, M.D., and Michelle B. Riba, M.D.,
Series Editors

Beginning with 1998, the annual Review of Psychiatry adopts a new format. What were individual sections bound together in a large volume will be published only as independent monographs. Each monograph provides an update on a particular topic. Readers may then selectively purchase those monographs of particular interest to them. Last year, Volume 16 was available in the large volume and individual monographs, and the individually published sections were immensely successful. We think this new format adds flexibility and convenience to the always popular series.

Our goal is to maintain the overall mission of this series—that is, to provide useful and current clinical information, linked to new research evidence. For 1998 we have selected topics that overlap and relate to each other: 1) Psychopathology and Violent Crime, 2) New Treatments for Chemical Addictions, 3) Psychological Trauma, 4) Biology of Personality Disorders, 5) Child Psychopharmacology, and 6) Interpersonal Psychotherapy. All of the editors and chapter authors are experts in their fields. The monographs capture the current state of knowledge and practice while providing guideposts to future lines of investigation.

We are indebted to Helen ("Sam") McGowan for her dedication and skill and to Linda Gacioch for all of her help. We are indebted to the American Psychiatric Press, Inc., under the leadership of Carol C. Nadelson, M.D., who has supported this important and valued review series. We thank Claire Reinburg, Pamela Harley, Ron McMillen, and the APPI staff for all their generous assistance.

Foreword

John C. Markowitz, M.D.

Interpersonal psychotherapy (IPT) is attracting continuing research and increasing clinical interest. This monograph of the Review of Psychiatry series highlights some of the important developments of IPT as a research intervention; a full review of all of its new directions would require a more encyclopedic volume. The first chapter documents current and likely future roles of IPT in clinical practice. The inclusion of IPT in the American Psychiatric Press Review of Psychiatry series suggests that it has been recognized as an important treatment of some Axis I disorders.

Like cognitive-behavioral therapy (CBT), IPT has gained popularity as a tested, focused treatment for specific psychiatric disorders. Its short-term efficacy has been demonstrated for a number of disorders. Economic pressures have also contributed to the burgeoning interest in empirically proven time-limited treatments. Developed in the 1970s as a research intervention, IPT has demonstrated efficacy for acute major depression in a series of randomized, controlled clinical trials. Its success in those studies has led to its adaptation and testing in the treatment of other diagnostic groups, including nonmood disorders. This series of presentations highlights some—but hardly all—recent research on the efficacy of IPT. The other important development in IPT is its recent translation from an almost purely research intervention into clinical practice.

Chapter 1, the overview of IPT by Myrna Weissman, Ph.D., and John Markowitz, M.D., reviews the breadth of IPT research and its clinical expansion. The succeeding chapters discuss particular adaptations of IPT in greater detail, reviewing exciting sequential steps in the application of IPT to particular patient populations. For each patient population, the indication of IPT has been tested in treatment studies. Some of these populations appear to be good targets for IPT: adolescents and HIV-positive patients, for example, may for different reasons prefer antidepressant psychotherapy to pharmacotherapy. For lack of space we have had to omit chapters on topics that might have equal value: for example, on IPT as a treatment for geriatric depression or for depressed patients in the primary care setting.

IPT has been successful in several landmark psychotherapy trials, including the acute National Institute of Mental Health (NIMH) Treatment of Depression Collaborative Research Program (TDCRP) and the Pittsburgh maintenance study of recurrent major depression. In addition to its use with various subtypes of mood disorders, including bipolar and dysthymic disorders, it has been tested as a treatment for bulimia (with good outcome) and substance abuse (with unsuccessful outcome). IPT has also been adapted to couples and group therapy formats, as a telephone intervention, and in a variant form for non–mental health workers (interpersonal counseling).

Increasing numbers of clinicians are training in IPT in residencies and continuing medical education programs in the United States and Canada. Interest in IPT is also growing abroad: its treatment manual has been translated into several languages, and trials are planned or under way in European countries.

In Chapter 2, Laura Mufson, Ph.D., and Donna Moreau, M.D., discuss the adaptation of IPT to treat depressed adolescent patients. This is an area of great interest and importance, since there has been only one positive controlled pharmacological trial of depression in this population. In collaboration with Myrna Weissman, Ph.D., the late Gerald L. Klerman, M.D., and Donna Moreau, M.D., Mufson developed and successfully tested this treatment in an open trial and a controlled treatment trial.

Cynthia Spanier, Ph.D., and Ellen Frank, Ph.D., describe in Chapter 3 the groundbreaking work on maintenance treatment of recurrent depression by the Pittsburgh group led by Ellen Frank, Ph.D., and David Kupfer, M.D. This study is the only long-term investigation of antidepressant prophylaxis using psychotherapy; it also added considerably to knowledge of the long-term pharmacotherapy of recurrent major depression. The investigators treated patients with highly recurrent major depression to remission using high-dosage imipramine and weekly IPT, stabilized remitters for several months, and then randomized them to five 3-year maintenance treatment conditions, three of which included a once-monthly maintenance form of IPT. Even this seemingly dilute form of IPT had a protective effect against relapse.

In Chapter 4, Christopher Fairburn, D.M., F.R.C.Psych., discusses the important studies he conducted in Oxford comparing IPT and CBT as treatments for bulimia in patients who were not clinically depressed. His results convinced this cognitive therapist of the efficacy of IPT, which worked as well as CBT and better than a behavioral control condition. The results also represented an important conceptual advance in demonstrating that IPT is efficacious in treating nonmood disorders.

Depression often accompanies physical illness. Holly Swartz, M.D., and John Markowitz, M.D., in Chapter 5 describe work at Cornell Medical College in New York adapting IPT for the treatment of depressed HIV-positive patients and testing this adaptation in a four-cell study similar to the NIMH TDCRP. IPT appeared to be an apt treatment for these patients facing life crises.

Chapter 1

An Overview of Interpersonal Psychotherapy

Myrna M. Weissman, Ph.D., and
John C. Markowitz, M.D.

Interpersonal psychotherapy (IPT) was developed in the 1970s as a time-limited treatment for major depression. IPT was defined in a manual and tested in randomized clinical trials by the late Gerald L. Klerman, M.D., and collaborators (1984). Its success in research trials led to its modification for subtypes of mood disorders as well as nonmood disorders (Klerman and Weissman 1993). IPT has also been adapted for use as a long-term treatment, in couples and group formats, as a telephone intervention, and in a patient self-help guide (Weissman 1995). A host of new research applications are being studied.

Having begun as a research intervention, IPT has only lately been disseminated among clinicians and in residency training programs. Requests for training in IPT have increased following IPT milestones such as the publication of efficacy data, the promulgation of practice guidelines that include IPT among antidepressant treatments, and its endorsement by *Consumers Guide* (1995). Managed care and economic pressures have also aroused growing interest in defined and proven treatments for managed

This material was adapted from Weissman MM, Markowitz JC: "Interpersonal Psychotherapy: Current Status." *Arch Gen Psychiatry* 51:599–606, 1994, and from Weissman MM, Markowitz JC: "Interpersonal Psychotherapy: Status 1997," in *Comprehensive Textbook of Psychiatry*, Vol 1, 8th Edition. Edited by Kaplan HI, Sadock BJ. Baltimore, Williams & Wilkins (in press).

This work was supported in part by Grant MH49635 from the National Institute of Mental Health and a fund established in the New York Community Trust by DeWitt-Wallace (Dr. Markowitz).

care. IPT has been translated into several languages and appears to be spreading in non-English-speaking countries.

In this chapter we briefly describe the concepts and techniques of IPT and its current status of adaptation, efficacy data, and training. We also provide a guide to developments and a reference list but not a comprehensive review. (For a complete description of the IPT method, see Klerman et al. 1984; for some of the adaptations, see the other chapters in this text and Klerman and Weissman 1993; and for the patient guide, see Weissman 1995.)

Practice Guidelines

In 1993 practice guidelines appeared for mental health professionals (Karasu et al. 1993) and primary care practitioners (Depression Guideline Panel 1993). The two sets of guidelines differ considerably in their scope, audience, and the level of scientific basis they require for treatment recommendation. Neither set of guidelines claims to define the standard of care for any individual patient. Each discusses IPT as an acute and maintenance treatment for depression, used alone or in combination with medication.

American Psychiatric Association Practice Guidelines

The American Psychiatric Association practice guidelines for major depression in adults (Karasu et al. 1993) cite IPT among other psychotherapies. The guidelines did not require efficacy data from controlled clinical trials as a criterion for inclusion. Karasu et al. (1993, p. 6) describe IPT as useful for patients in the "midst of recent conflicts with significant others and for those having difficulty adjusting to an altered career or social role or other life transition." The evidence we provide in this chapter suggests that these are minimal, conservative indications, although many patients do present with such recent life changes.

Primary Care Guidelines

The clinical practice guidelines for treatment of depression in primary care settings are more extensive, comprising four volumes (Depression Guideline Panel 1993). Both the physician and patient guides list IPT, cognitive-behavioral therapy (CBT), behavioral, brief dynamic, and marital therapy as treatments for depression. IPT is recommended as an acute treatment of nonpsychotic depression: to remove symptoms, prevent relapse and recurrence, correct causal psychological problems with secondary symptom resolution, and correct secondary consequences of depression. The guidelines state that medication alone may be sufficient to prevent relapse or recurrence and to maintain remitted patients with recurrent depression (Frank et al. 1990).

The guidelines describe IPT, CBT, and behavioral treatments as "effective in most cases of mild-to-moderate depression" (Depression Guideline Panel 1993, Vol. 2, p. 12), but indications "for continuation phase psychotherapy are unclear," even though "two studies are suggestive that continuation psychotherapy may reduce the relapse rate" (Depression Guideline Panel 1993, Vol. 2, p. 18). The patient guidelines list behavioral, cognitive, and IPT as the "most well-studied [sic] for their effectiveness in reducing symptoms of major depressive disorder" (Depression Guideline Panel 1993, Vol. 4, p. 23).

Overview of IPT

Efficacy studies of psychotherapy as a treatment for depression and other disorders have been reviewed in several publications (e.g., Jarrett and Rush 1994; Klerman et al. 1994). IPT was initially formulated as a time-limited, weekly outpatient treatment for depressed patients (Klerman et al. 1984). Based on the ideas of the interpersonal school (Sullivan 1953) but making no etiological assumptions, IPT uses the connection between onset of depressive symptoms and current interpersonal problems as a pragmatic treatment focus. IPT deals with current rather than past interpersonal relationships, focusing on the patient's immediate social context. The IPT therapist attempts to intervene in symptom formation and social dysfunction associated with depression rather than addressing enduring aspects of personality. Personality is in any case hard to assess during an episode of an Axis I disorder such as depression.

Phases of Treatment

As an acute treatment, IPT has three phases. The first, usually encompassing one to three sessions, includes diagnostic evaluation and psychiatric history and sets the framework for the treatment. The therapist reviews symptoms, diagnoses the patient as depressed by standard criteria (American Psychiatric Association 1994), and gives the patient the sick role (Parsons 1951). The sick role may excuse the patient from overwhelming social obligations but requires the patient to work in treatment to recover full function. The psychiatric history includes the "interpersonal inventory," a review of the patient's current social functioning and close relationships and their patterns and mutual expectations. Changes in relationships proximal to the onset of symptoms, such as death of a loved one, children leaving home, worsening marital strife, or isolation from a confidant, are elucidated. This review provides a framework for understanding the social and interpersonal context of the onset of depressive symptoms and defines the focus of treatment.

Having assessed the need for medication based on symptom severity, past history and response to treatment, and patient preference, the therapist educates the patient about depression by explicitly discussing the diagnosis, including the constellation of symptoms that define major depression, and what the patient might expect from treatment. The therapist next links the depressive syndrome to the patient's interpersonal situation in a formulation (Markowitz and Swartz 1997) that uses as a framework one of four interpersonal problem areas: 1) grief, 2) interpersonal role disputes, 3) role transitions, or 4) interpersonal deficits.

In the middle phase, the therapist pursues strategies specific to the chosen interpersonal problem area, as described in the manual (Klerman et al. 1984). For *grief*, defined as complicated bereavement following the death of a loved one, the therapist facilitates the catharsis of mourning and gradually helps the patient to find new activities and relationships to compensate for the loss. *Role disputes* are conflicts with a significant other: a spouse or other family members, co-worker, or close friend. The therapist helps the patient explore the relationship, the nature of the dispute, whether it has reached an impasse, and options to resolve it. If these measures fail, they may conclude that the relationship has reached an impasse and consider ways to circumvent the impasse or to end the relationship. *Role transition* includes change in life status, such as beginning or ending a relationship or career, moving, promotion, retirement, graduation, or diagnosis of a medical illness. The patient learns to deal with the change by recognizing positive and negative aspects of the new role he or she is assuming and assets and liabilities of the old role being replaced. *Interpersonal deficits*, the residual fourth IPT problem area, defines the patient as lacking social skills, including having problems in initiating or sustaining relationships.

IPT sessions address present, here-and-now problems rather than childhood or developmental issues. Sessions open with the question: "How have things been since we last met?" This inquiry focuses the patient on recent interpersonal events and recent mood, which the therapist helps the patient to link. Therapists take an active, nonneutral, supportive, and hopeful stance to counter the depressed patient's pessimism. They emphasize the options that exist for change in the patient's life, options that the depression may have kept the patient from seeing or exploring fully.

The final phase of IPT, occupying the last few of the 12–16 weeks of treatment, supports the patient's newly regained sense of independence and competence by recognizing and consolidating therapeutic gains. The therapist also helps the patient to anticipate and develop ways of identifying and countering depressive symptoms should they arise in the future.

Use of IPT in Mood Disorders

IPT is one of the most carefully studied psychotherapies for mood disorders, and the only psychotherapy tested in a maintenance treatment study (see Chapter 3).

Acute Treatment of Major Depression

The efficacy of IPT as an acute antidepressant treatment was first tested in a four-cell, 16-week randomized trial comparing IPT, amitriptyline (AMI), their combination, and a nonscheduled control treatment for 81 outpatients with major depression (DiMascio et al. 1979; Weissman et al. 1979). No significant difference appeared between IPT and AMI in symptom reduction at the end of treatment, although AMI alleviated symptoms more quickly. Each active treatment more effectively reduced symptoms than did the nonscheduled control group, and combined AMI and IPT was more effective than either active monotherapy. Naturalistic follow-up at 1 year found that many patients sustained benefits from the brief IPT intervention, and patients who received IPT developed significantly better psychosocial functioning, whether or not they received medication. This effect on social function was not found for AMI alone and had not been evident for IPT at the end of the 16-week trial (Weissman et al. 1981). Many patients across treatments, however, reported requiring additional treatment over the follow-up year. This finding suggested that acute treatment did not "cure" depression, a fact now recognized in many studies that include a maintenance phase.

The multisite National Institute of Mental Health Treatment of Depression Collaborative Research Program (NIMH TDCRP) (Elkin et al. 1989) is the most ambitious acute treatment study to date. Investigators randomly assigned 250 depressed outpatients to 16 weeks of IPT, CBT, or either imipramine (IMI) or placebo plus clinical management. Most subjects completed at least 15 weeks or 12 treatment sessions. Less symptomatic patients— those with a 17-item Hamilton Rating Scale for Depression (Hamilton 1960) score of 19 or less—improved in all treatments, including placebo. Among more severely depressed patients, IMI worked most rapidly and was most consistently superior to placebo. IPT was comparable to IMI on several outcome measures, including the Hamilton Rating Scale for Depression, and showed a mean outcome superior to placebo for the more severely depressed patients. CBT was not superior to placebo for this group.

Klein and Ross (1993) reanalyzed the NIMH TDCRP efficacy data. The Johnson-Neyman technique produced an ordering for treatment efficacy with "medication superior to psychotherapy, [and] the psychotherapies somewhat superior to placebo . . . particularly among the symptomatic and impaired patients" (Klein and Ross 1993, p. 241). The authors found "CBT relatively inferior to IPT for patients with BDI [Beck Depression Inventory] scores greater than approximately 30, generally considered the boundary between moderate and severe depression" (p. 247). The reanalysis is fairly consistent with results reported by Elkin et al. (1989) but sharpens differences among treatments.

In an 18-month naturalistic follow-up study of TDCRP subjects, Shea et al. (1992) found no significant difference in recovery among remitters (defined by the presence of minimal or no symptoms following the end of treatment, sustained during follow-up) among the four treatment groups. Of the subjects who had acutely remitted, 30% of CBT, 26% of IPT, 19% of IMI, and 20% of placebo subjects remained in remission during that time span. Among remitters at the end of the 16 weeks, relapse over the 18-month follow-up was 36% for CBT, 33% for IPT, 50% for IMI, and 33% for placebo. The authors concluded that 16 weeks of specific treatments were insufficient to achieve full and lasting recovery for many patients.

Hoencamp (E. Hoencamp and M. Blom, personal communication, October 1997) and colleagues are undertaking a study of IPT versus nefazodone, alone and in combination, for the acute treatment of major depression in the Hague, the Netherlands.

Predictors of Response

Large comparative treatment studies such as the TDCRP and the Pittsburgh maintenance study allow the exploration of patient and therapist characteristics that may contribute to treatment outcome. Sotsky and colleagues (1991), analyzing the TDCRP results, found that patients with low baseline levels of social dysfunction responded well to IPT, whereas those with severe social deficits (probably equivalent to the interpersonal deficits problem area) responded less well. Patients with greater symptom severity and difficulty in concentrating responded poorly to CBT. High initial severity of depression and impairment of functioning predicted superior response to IPT and to IMI. IMI also worked most efficaciously for patients with difficulty functioning at work—perhaps reflecting its faster onset of action.

In subsequent analyses, Sotsky (1997) reported that TDCRP subjects with symptoms of atypical depression, in particular mood reactivity and reversed neurovegetative symptoms (hypersomnia, hyperphagia, or weight gain) responded poorly to IMI but well to IPT and CBT. This outcome is consistent with previous research findings that tricyclic antidepressants are a suboptimal treatment option for atypical depression. Barber and Muenz (1996) reexamined the TDCRP data. Looking only at subjects who completed treatment, they found that IPT was more efficacious than CBT for patients with obsessive personality disorder, whereas CBT was better for avoidant personality disorder on the Hamilton Rating Scale for Depression. In contrast, Blatt and colleagues (1995) used a different measure, the Dysfunctional Attitude Scale (Weissman and Beck 1978), to measure the similar concepts of perfectionism and need for approval among subjects from the TDCRP but did not find significant results. Neither approach used definitive diagnostic measures for personality disorder. The role of personality traits on depressive outcome in IPT remains of great interest and clearly requires further study.

In Pittsburgh, Thase and colleagues (1997) found that depressed patients with abnormal electroencephalogram (EEG) sleep profiles (sleep efficiency, rapid eye movement [REM] latency, and REM density) responded significantly more poorly to IPT than did patients with undisturbed sleep parameters. This finding was not an artifact of symptom severity. Three-quarters of the IPT nonresponders subsequently responded to antidepressant medication. Meanwhile, Frank and colleagues (1991) found that the "purity" of IPT—the ability of the therapist to keep sessions focused on interpersonal themes—was significantly correlated with prevention of relapse in their maintenance study of IPT for recurrent major depression (see Chapter 3). Patients whose monthly IPT maintenance sessions had high interpersonal specificity survived a mean 2 years before developing depression, whereas those whose therapy had a low interpersonal focus were afforded only 5 months of protection before relapse.

Continuation or Maintenance Treatment

IPT was first developed and tested in an 8-month, six-cell trial (Klerman et al. 1974; Paykel et al. 1975). This study would be considered today a continuation rather than a maintenance treatment, since the concept of long-term treatment of depression has changed. Acutely depressed female outpatients ($N = 150$) who responded (>50% symptom reduction rated by a clinical interviewer) to a 4- to 6-week acute phase of AMI were randomized to receive 8 months of treatment with *weekly* IPT alone, AMI alone, combined IPT and AMI, IPT and placebo alone, or no pill. Randomization to IPT or a low contact condition occurred at entry into the continuation phase, whereas randomization to medication, placebo, or no pill occurred at the end of the second month of continuation. Maintenance pharmacotherapy was found to prevent relapse and symptom exacerbation, whereas IPT improved social functioning (Weissman et al. 1974). The effects of IPT on social functioning were not apparent for 6–8 months. No negative treatment interactions were found, and combined psychotherapy-pharmacotherapy had the best outcome.

In the longest—and only—maintenance trial of psychotherapy for prophylaxis of depression, Frank et al. (1991) studied 128 outpatients with multiply recurrent depression (see also Frank 1991b; Frank et al. 1989). This important research, which demonstrated the benefits of even a monthly dosage for patients at high risk for relapse, is described in Chapter 3. The finding of an

82-week survival time without recurrence with IPT alone would suffice to protect many women with recurrent depression through pregnancy and nursing without medication. Further study is required to determine whether the efficacy of IPT differs in relation to newer medications (e.g., selective serotonin reuptake inhibitors). The effectiveness of more frequent than monthly IPT needs to be addressed. A study of differing doses of maintenance IPT for depressed patients is under way in Pittsburgh.

Geriatric Depressed Patients

The first use of IPT in geriatric depressed patients added it to a 6-week medication trial in order to enhance compliance and to provide some treatment in the placebo control group (Rothblum et al. 1982; Sholomskas et al. 1983). Noting that grief and role transition specific to life changes were the prime foci of treatment, the authors suggested IPT modifications including more flexible duration of sessions, greater use of practical advice and support (e.g., arranging transportation and calling the physician), and recognition that major role changes may be impractical and detrimental (e.g., divorce at age 75).

A 6-week clinical trial comparing IPT with nortriptyline in 30 geriatric depressed patients showed some advantages for IPT, which were largely due to medication side effects that produce higher attrition in the medication group (Sloane et al. 1985). IPT was not modified for this study.

A 3-year maintenance study of geriatric patients with recurrent depression in Pittsburgh is using a design similar to that of the Frank et al. (1990) study. The investigators modified IPT for geriatric patients, calling it IPT–Late Life Maintenance (IPT-LLM) treatment. During the acute phase patients received combined nortriptyline and IPT (Reynolds et al. 1996). The study then compared IPT-LLM alone, nortriptyline alone, IPT-LLM and nortriptyline, IPT-LLM and placebo, and placebo alone as randomized discontinuation maintenance therapies (Reynolds et al. 1992). The manual has been modified to allow more flexible length of sessions, since elderly patients may not tolerate 50-minute sessions. Some of the authors found that older patients need to address early life relationships in their psychotherapy, a distinction from the typical here-and-now focus of IPT. Like Sholomskas et al. (1983), Reynolds et al. (1992) found that therapists needed to help patients solve practical problems and should share awareness that some problems may not be amenable to resolutions, such as existential late life issues or lifelong psychopathology (Rothblum et al. 1982; Sholomskas et al. 1983). Preliminary results showed that elderly depressed patients whose sleep quality normalized by early continuation of treatment had an 80% chance of remaining well during the first year of maintenance treatment. The response rate was similar in patients receiving nortriptyline or IPT (Reynolds et al. 1997).

Bereavement-Related Depression

An ongoing study in Pittsburgh compares IPT with nortriptyline for acute treatment of bereavement-related major depression (C. F. Reynolds, personal communication, 1996). The IPT modification includes more detailed information gathering in the initial phase of treatment on the quality of earlier and current relationships and roles and determines available social supports for spousal bereavement. Detailed information on practical quality of life issues include, for example, bill payment, financial burden, leisure activities, and children (see Miller and Silberman 1996 and Miller et al. 1994 for adaptations).

Depressed Adolescents

Mufson et al. (1993) modified IPT to incorporate adolescent developmental issues (IPT-A), adding as a fifth problem area the single-parent family, an interpersonal situation found frequently among their adolescents. Mufson and colleagues (1993, 1994; Moreau et al. 1991) have tested this approach in both an open trial and a controlled clinical trial (see Chapter 2).

Depressed Adolescent Mothers

L. A. Gillies and colleagues, at the Clarke Institute, Toronto, Canada, are completing a pilot study of depressed pregnant adolescents (ages 15–19). Thirty patients, all scoring 14 or higher on the Beck Depression Inventory (BDI) (Beck 1978), were randomly assigned to 12 weekly sessions of arts and crafts, a psychoeducational group, or individual IPT. Eleven subjects terminated early, with attrition approximately equal across groups. Results are pending.

Depressed HIV-Positive Patients

Markowitz et al. (1992) modified IPT for depressed human immunodeficiency virus (HIV) patients (IPT-HIV), emphasizing common issues among this population, including concern about illness and death, grief, and role transitions. In a pilot open trial, 21 of the 24 depressed patients responded with symptom reduction. A 16-week trial randomized 101 subjects to IPT-HIV, CBT, supportive psychotherapy (SP), and IMI plus SP (Markowitz et al., in press). As with the more depressed subjects in the TDCRP study (Elkin et al. 1989), IPT and IMI plus SP resulted in the greatest improvement (see Chapter 5).

Depressed Primary Care Patients

Schulberg and colleagues completed a clinical trial comparing IPT with pharmacotherapy for depressed ambulatory medical patients in a primary care setting (Schulberg and Scott 1991; Schulberg et al. 1993). The IPT manual was not modified, but IPT conformed with practices of the primary care center (e.g., nurses took vital signs before each session). If a patient was medically hospitalized, IPT continued in the hospital when possible.

Patients with current major depression ($N = 276$) were assigned to either IPT, nortriptyline, or primary care physicians' usual care. They were treated with IPT weekly for 16 weeks and monthly thereafter for 4 months (Schulberg et al. 1996). Depressive symptoms improved more rapidly with either nortriptyline or IPT than with usual primary care. Among treatment completers, approximately 70% who received nortriptyline or IPT, but only 20% who received usual primary care, were judged recovered at 8 months. Brown et al. (1996) found that patients with lifetime comorbid panic disorder, compared with major depression alone, had poorer recovery regardless of treatment.

Conjoint IPT for Depressed Patients With Marital Disputes

Since marital conflict, separation, and divorce have been associated with onset and course of depressive episodes (Rounsaville et al. 1979), and individual psychotherapy for depressed patients in marital disputes may lead to premature termination of some marriages (Gurman and Kniskern 1978), a manual was developed for conjoint therapy of depressed patients with marital disputes (IPT-CM) (Klerman and Weissman 1993). IPT-CM focuses on the current marital dispute and involves the spouse in all sessions. Eighteen patients with major depression linked to the onset or exacerbation of marital disputes were randomly assigned to 16 weeks of individual IPT or IPT-CM. Patients in both treatments showed the same reduction in depressive symptoms. Patients treated following IPT-CM guidelines had significantly better marital adjustment, greater marital affection, and better sexual relations than did patients treated with IPT alone (Foley et al. 1989). These preliminary findings require replication with a larger sample and other control groups.

Antepartum and Postpartum Depression

M. G. Spinelli at Columbia University is using IPT to treat women with antepartum depression. Examination of this role transition focuses on the depressed pregnant woman's self-evaluation as a parent, physiological changes of pregnancy, and altered relationships with spouse or significant other and other children. Spinelli has added a fifth interpersonal problem area, complicated pregnancy. Timing and duration of sessions require flexibility because of bed rest, delivery, obstetrical complications, and child care. Young children may be brought to sessions and breast-fed by postpartum mothers. Telephone sessions and hospital visits are sometimes necessary. Spinelli is undertaking a controlled clinical trial comparing IPT with a didactic parent education group in depressed pregnant women over 16 weeks of acute treatment and six monthly follow-up sessions.

Swartz and colleagues (1997) at Cornell Medical Center evaluated IPT in a small pilot study for depressed, pregnant, HIV-positive patients. S. Stuart and M. W. O'Hara (personal communication, May 1996) are currently comparing IPT with a waiting list control for women with postpartum depression. They assess both the mothers' symptom states and interactions with their infants.

Dysthymic Disorder

In a modification of IPT for dysthymic disorder (IPT-D), patients are encouraged to reconceptualize what they have seen as their lifelong character flaws as ego-dystonic, chronic mood-dependent symptoms: as chronic "state" rather than "trait." Contrary to expectation, open treatment found that dysthymic patients with lifelong chronicity had a reduction of depressive symptoms in 16 weekly IPT sessions. Markowitz (1994, 1997) treated a total of 16 pilot subjects: none worsened, and 11 remitted. Medication benefits roughly half of dysthymic patients (Kocsis et al. 1988; Thase et al. 1996), but nonresponders may need psychotherapy, and even medication responders may benefit from combined treatment (Markowitz 1994). Based on these pilot results, a comparative study of 16 weeks of IPT-D alone, SP, sertraline plus clinical management, and a combined IPT and sertraline cell is under way at Cornell Medical Center.

G. Browne, M. Steiner, and others at McMaster University in Hamilton, Canada, are studying some 700 dysthymic patients receiving unmodified IPT or sertraline alone or in combination for 1 year. They will compare variable doses of IPT (G. Browne, personal communication, 1996). A trial under way in Toronto is comparing IPT with the short-term psychodynamic therapy of Luborsky (1984) in 72 patients who meet criteria for dysthymia with or without major depression (double depression). Patients receive 12 weekly sessions followed by four monthly sessions (L. A. Gillies, personal communication, August 1995). Initial results of IPT treatment indicate that most patients reported a reduction of symptoms (Frey and L. A. Gillies, personal communication, 1996). The authors found that dysthymic patients responded to IPT, similar to patients with major depression, but that the long-standing nature of their illness made dysthymic patients more difficult to treat.

Bipolar Disorder

Ehlers and colleagues (1988) in Pittsburgh are assessing the benefits for bipolar patients of adjunctive IPT (IPT-BP) modified by social zeitgeber theory—behavioral scheduling of daily and sleep patterns—as maintenance treatment of lithium-stabilized bipolar patients. Comparing IPT-BP with medication alone (Frank 1991a), the 3-year maintenance treatment study will initially include biweekly IPT visits, tapering to monthly sessions in the final 2 years.

Use of IPT in Other Disorders

The success of IPT in treating mood disorders has led to its application to nonmood syndromes as well.

Substance Abuse

IPT has not demonstrated efficacy in two clinical trials with substance-abusing patients. The first study found no additional benefit in reducing psychopathology for adjunctive IPT added to standard treatment, compared with the standard program alone, for 72 methadone-maintained opiate abusers (Rounsaville et al. 1983). The same team in a separate trial found 12 weeks of IPT ineffective and marginally worse than behavioral treatment for 42 cocaine abusers attempting to achieve abstinence (Carroll et al. 1991). The two negative studies suggest limits to the utility of IPT but do not necessarily preclude its use for treating substance abuse. IPT might be useful, for example, in the treatment of newly abstinent alcohol-dependent patients, who face numerous psychosocial stressors that have been shown to precipitate relapse.

Bulimia

Fairburn et al. (1991, 1993, 1995) altered IPT for two studies of bulimic patients. This research showed IPT to have long-term benefits comparable to CBT and superior to a behavioral control condition. For a fuller discussion of this first successful adaptation of IPT to a nonmood disorder, see Chapter 4.

Group Format for Bulimia

Drawing on the work of Fairburn, Wilfley et al. (1993) modified IPT in a group format of 16 weekly sessions and compared it with group CBT and a waiting list control (WL) for 56 women with nonpurging bulimia. At termination, patients treated with IPT group format for bulimia (IPT-G) and CBT each showed significantly reduced binge eating, whereas WL controls did not. These results persisted at 1-year follow-up. A randomized clinical trial of 162 women is now comparing group IPT and CBT for 20 sessions over 20 weeks. The initial IPT phase, in which the therapist identifies the problem area and presents IPT concepts and the treatment contract, is conducted individually. Groups meet for 90 minutes.

Social Phobia

Unlike CBT, IPT has not been tested in controlled trials for the treatment of anxiety disorders. The interpersonal aspects of social phobia make it a natural starting place for such research. IPT is being modified for social phobia independently by Lipsitz at Columbia and by S. Stuart and M. W. O'Hara at the University of Iowa, with open trials in progress at both sites. J. Lipsitz (personal communication, September 1996), having completed nine pilot cases, reports that the standard IPT ingredients, including the medical model, provision of the sick role, and supportive therapeutic stance, appear to benefit most patients. The interpersonal formulation, a linking of anxiety symptoms to interpersonal context, appeals more to some patients than to others. A patient with prominent blushing, for example, attributed her social anxiety to the blushing, insisting it was unrelated to her interactions with other people or her ability to express emotion freely; nonetheless, IPT seemed to help her.

Social phobic patients often present in role transitions: geographic moves, career changes, separations from significant others, or the onset of a major illness. Social anxiety may increase in intensity or may simply pose a greater problem in the context of these transitions. Because social phobia often has an early onset and chronic course, lacking acute precipitants, Lipsitz borrowed an approach from Markowitz (1993, 1997) on IPT for dysthymic disorder. By providing the medical model of social phobia, offering reassurance that the patient has a disorder that is treatable, and instilling hope for change, the therapist initiates a "therapeutic role transition." The patient recognizes shyness, passivity, and social awkwardness as symptoms of a disorder rather than his or her true personality. This formulation creates a positive stressor, which serves as a basis for exploring current interpersonal experiences ("It sounds like you can be quite assertive with your staff now that you are not letting the social phobia get in the way").

S. Stuart (personal communication, May 1996) notes two groups of socially phobic patients: those with avoidant features who desire relationships but have difficulty maintaining them and those with schizoid traits who want to minimize social interactions. The latter seek treatment only when circumstances require them to interact more frequently. An example was a librarian with no psychiatric history who sought treatment upon receiving a promotion. Her new job required supervising other employees, whereas before she had contentedly shelved and cataloged books with minimal social contact. Addressing this career change as a role transition helped the patient through the acute stress, although Stuart was skeptical of the long-term benefit of treatment.

Social Phobia in a Group Format

M. M. Weissman and B. Jacobson (unpublished data) have adapted IPT in a group format for patients with shyness. The patients had social phobia in unstructured interpersonal situations: at parties and in intimate discussions with significant others but not in defined work situations. Most patients were successful in professional or business careers despite their phobias.

The 10-session, time-limited group focused on defining and describing the diagnosis, giving the patient the sick role, and finding practical strategies for dealing with shyness in specific situations (e.g., developing scripts to initiate a more personal conversation with an estranged father or a discussion with a spouse about having a baby). As noted by Lipsitz, the chronicity of the disorder led to a focus on a therapeutic role transition from an impaired to less-impaired state. The group format seemed to provide a safe haven for patients to interact with others who had similar symptoms.

Panic Disorder

A manual for IPT in panic disorder is being developed by A. Arzt and M. van Rijsoort in Maastricht, the Netherlands.

Body Dysmorphic Disorder

H. Veale is conducting a 15-week clinical trial in London comparing CBT with IPT for patients with body dysmorphic disorder, preoccupation with an imagined defect in appearance that causes distress in social functioning.

Chronic Somatization in Primary Care Patients

Scott and Ikkos (1996) have modified IPT to manage patients with chronic somatization in primary care. This adaptation adds a fifth problem area, the patient's relationship with health professionals and the pursuit of medical care. J. Scott (personal communication, 1996) notes that the IPT medical model works readily with these patients because of their inappropriate use of the health care system. Treatment seeking is reconceived as an interpersonal issue. These patients are easily recruited for IPT treatment. Scott and Ikkos note that 12 sessions may be insufficient to engage patients and develop a working alliance. The therapist emphasizes that he or she is not trying to modify the patient's experience of "pain" but rather wants to help the patient deal more effectively with the problem. An open trial of 20–30 patients is planned.

Borderline Personality Disorder

In Toronto, L. A. Gillies has adapted IPT for patients with borderline personality disorder. The focus in the initial phase is on assessment of symptom patterns related to the disorder, such as anger and impulsivity in interpersonal relations (Angus and Gillies 1994). A fifth problem area, self-image, has been added to address the identity disturbance that is central to borderline personality disorder. Telephone contact is used during crises but not encouraged in lieu of regular scheduled sessions. A pilot randomized trial on 24 patients is under way comparing 12 weekly sessions of IPT with relationship management therapy, with monthly follow-up for 6 months. The trial uses a sequential treatment–therapist crossover design to control for therapist effects.

Initial results show lower attrition in IPT (10%) than in the control group (50%). Comparison of pre- and posttreatment scores of IPT patients with borderline personality and those with dysthymic or double depression found similar and significant symptomatic improvement across diagnostic groups (L. A. Gillies and Frey, personal communication). It will be interesting to see whether time-limited psychotherapy alleviates a time-resistant disorder such as borderline personality.

Other Applications

A modification of IPT for patients with insomnia has been developed by K. Müller-Popkens and G. Hajak (1996) in Hamburg, Germany. This research arose from the observation that insomnia is often associated with stressful interpersonal life events. The approach emphasizes management of insomnia and the regularizing of social rhythms adapted from the work of Frank (1991a) with bipolar patients. The initial phase presents information on sleep hygiene and rhythm, and patients keep a sleep diary.

IPT is being delivered over the telephone to housebound patients with metastatic breast cancer by J. Donnelly, J. Holland, and others at Memorial Sloan-Kettering Cancer Center in New York. A similar study is under way at Clarke Institute, Toronto (L. A. Gillies, personal communication, 1996).

Stuart and Cole (1996) have modified IPT for patients with depression status after myocardial infarction. The adaptation includes careful initial medical evaluation to ensure that insomnia, anergia, and other vegetative symptoms represent clinical depression rather than cardiac illness. Stuart notes that care must be taken to ensure that the physical symptoms exceed those expected during this convalescent period. IPT confronts grief over loss of the healthy state and struggles with mortality, remorse over past unhealthy behavior, and the effects of the illness on marital relations and work. Another theme for many patients is being forced into the passive role of receiving care after a life of independence. No other trials of counseling with patients after myocardial infarction have focused on depression (Stuart and Cole 1996). Stuart and Cole report that although these patients acknowledge depression, they often refuse psychological intervention, even if treatment is labeled as stress reduction or coping skills development.

Interpersonal Counseling

Distress

Many patients presenting to primary care practices report psychiatric symptoms yet do not meet full criteria for a psychiatric disorder. Their symptoms can be debilitating and result in fruitless "million-dollar workups" and high utilization of medical procedures (Wells et al. 1989). Interpersonal counseling (IPC), based on IPT, was designed for distressed primary care patients who do not meet syndromal criteria for psychiatric disorders. IPC is administered by health care professionals, usually nurse practitioners without formal psychiatric training, for a maximum of six sessions. The first session can last as long as 30 minutes; subsequent sessions are briefer.

IPC therapists assess the patient's current functioning, recent life events, occupational and familial stress, and changes in interpersonal relationships. They assume that such events may provide the context in which emotional and bodily symptoms occur. Patients ($N = 128$) presenting to a primary care clinic and scoring 6 or higher on the Goldberg General Health Questionnaire (GHQ) (Goldberg 1972) were randomized to either IPC or usual care without psychological treatment (Klerman et al. 1987). Over an average of 3 months, often involving only one to two IPC sessions, IPC subjects showed significantly greater symptom relief than controls on the GHQ, particularly an improvement in depressed mood. IPC led to greater use of mental health services by patients newly attuned to the psychological source of their symptoms.

Subsyndromally Depressed Hospitalized Elderly Patients

Observing that depressive symptoms that did not reach criteria for major depression nonetheless impeded recovery of hospitalized elderly patients, Mossey et al. (1996) conducted a 10-session trial of IPC for elderly hospitalized medical patients with depressive symptoms. They modified IPC by increasing the number of sessions from 6 to 10, their duration from 30 to 60 minutes, and the flexibility of scheduling from once weekly to a schedule that reflected the patient's medical status. They randomized 76 hospitalized patients over age 60 who did not meet criteria for major depression but had depressive symptoms on two consecutive assessments to receive either IPC administered by clinical nurse specialists or usual care (UC). Researchers also followed a nondepressed control group. Patients found IPC feasible and acceptable. Assessment at 3 months showed nonsignificantly greater reduction in depressive symptoms and greater improvement on all outcome variables for IPC relative to UC versus a slight symptomatic increase among controls. Rehospitalization in the IPC and nondepressed control groups was virtually identical (11%–15%) and significantly less than the subsyndromally depressed group receiving usual care (50%). At 6 months, differences between IPC and UC groups reached statistical significance on reduction of depressive symptoms and self-rated health but not on physical or social functioning. A 1-year evaluation is pending. The investigators felt that 10 sessions were insufficient for some patients and that a maintenance phase might have been useful. They judged the clinical nurse specialists acceptable therapists.

Fried, Pelcovitz, and Kochen (personal communication, 1996) at North Shore University Hospital, Manhasset, New York, completed a 6-week open IPC trial with 30 mothers or caretakers of children with cancer. IPC was administered by a clinical psychologist and focused on the mother's functioning and adaptation to the child's illness.

IPC by Telephone

Because many patients avoid or have difficulty reaching an office for face-to-face treatment, IPC is being tested as a telephone treatment. An open trial under way at Memorial Sloan-Kettering Cancer Center in New York offers IPT to severely medically, but not psychiatrically, ill patients with metastatic breast cancer who are receiving high-dose chemotherapy. Both the patient and partner receive weekly 30-minute sessions for approximately 15 weeks. All patients have metastatic breast cancer considered incurable by standard treatments. Their chemotherapy regimen is unusually disabling, and patients must move to within minutes of the hospital for the 2–3 months of treatment, causing major disruptions for themselves and their families. They must take extended leaves from jobs and leave children and/or spouses at home. The purpose of the study was to adapt IPT to relieve cancer-related stress rather than depression, but the prevalence of depression and depressive symptoms is high. The investigators report that IPT fits a wide range of the patients' needs well. (Kornbluth, Donnelly, and Holland, personal communication, 1996).

Another pilot telephone trial under way is comparing IPT with no treatment in a naturalistic longitudinal study (M. M. Weissman and L. Miller, personal communication, 1996) of 30 patients who have had recurrent depression but have not received regular treatment.

IPT Patient Guide

Weissman (1995) has developed a user-friendly IPT patient guide with accompanying worksheets designed for patients who want to learn about or are receiving IPT. It leads the patient through treatment in simple language. Worksheets can be used to facilitate sessions or to monitor problem areas after treatment. Testing to determine whether the patient book facilitates treatment has not been undertaken. Informal reports by L. A. Gillies and J. C. Markowitz (personal communication, August 1996) note that patient response has been positive and that some therapists have found the patient guide useful during training in IPT.

Translations

IPT has been translated into Italian by Ceroni (see Klerman et al. 1989), into German by Schramm (1996), and into Japanese by

Ono (1997). Descriptions of IPT have appeared in Spanish (Puig 1995) and Dutch (Blom et al. 1996).

Training in IPT

Until recently, IPT practitioners were few and limited almost exclusively to participants in research studies. IPT training is now increasingly included in professional workshops and conferences, with training courses conducted at university centers in Canada, Europe, Asia, and New Zealand. A training videotape (Kingsley Communications, Houston, Texas) describes IPT and demonstrates the initial assessment phase of treatment.

Training workshops for mental health professionals from a variety of disciplines have been held by Markowitz at Cornell Medical School, New York; C. Cornes at the University of Pittsburgh; and L. A. Gillies in Toronto, Canada. IPT is taught in some but not most residency training programs (Markowitz 1995) and has been included in family practice and primary care training (L. A. Gillies, personal communication, 1996). IPT clinics have been established at the Clarke Institute in Toronto and at New York Hospital–Cornell Medical Center in New York City.

Although the principles of IPT are straightforward, training is more involved than simply reading the manual (Rounsaville et al. 1988; Weissman et al. 1982). Candidates should have a graduate clinical degree (M.D., Ph.D., M.S.W., or R.N.) and several years of experience conducting psychotherapy. IPT training programs are designed to help experienced therapists refocus their treatment by learning new techniques, not to teach novices psychotherapy. The training used in the TDCRP (Elkin et al. 1989) has become a model for subsequent research studies. This training includes a brief didactic phase, reviewing the manual, and a longer practicum during which the therapist treats two to three patients under close supervision monitored by videotapes of the sessions (Chevron and Rounsaville 1983). Rounsaville et al. (1986) found that psychotherapists who performed well on a first supervised IPT case often did not require further intensive supervision and that experienced therapists committed to the approach required less supervision than others (Rounsaville et al. 1988).

Conclusion

Evidence from controlled clinical trials suggests that IPT is a reasonable alternative or adjunct to medication as an acute, continuation, and maintenance treatment for patients with major depression; for acutely depressed HIV-positive and other medically ill patients; and for patients with bulimia. It is a promising, but still not fully tested, treatment for depressed adolescent and geriatric patients, dysthymic patients, primary care patients with mild depression, and depressed patients with marital disputes (as a couples treatment). More efficacy data are needed before stronger claims can be made. Open trials are encouraging but cannot be considered evidence of efficacy. IPT is not effective, compared with standard treatment, for opiate- and cocaine-addicted patients. Several IPT clinical trials are under way or planned based on modified treatment manuals, and several manuals are being developed. The manuals differ in the depth of their modifications, and some adaptations for particular disorders have not been formalized. There is little agreement on what a manualized IPT adaptation should include.

We view the development of psychotherapy manuals as progress. They will meet growing requests from third-party payers, managed care, and patients for accountability and specification of treatment. Manuals are a necessary first step for testing efficacy. Psychiatric and other mental health treatment training programs should include clinical instruction in time-limited, manual-defined psychotherapies in addition to exposing trainees to long-term psychotherapy. To our knowledge, there is no currently accepted model psychotherapy curriculum.

For experienced therapists, although IPT training programs are still not widely available, access is growing. The established training criteria for research have produced reliable therapists for clinical trials. Yet the educational process for IPT in clinical practice requires further study. What educational level and experience does a clinician need to learn IPT? How much supervision does an experienced therapist require?

IPT research to date has focused largely on outcome. With some effective outcomes now demonstrated, process research is worthwhile to determine specific ingredients of the treatment. Dismantling studies might be useful. For example, we consider the initial diagnostic and assessment phase of IPT essential to the clinical management of *all* depressed patients. The efficacy of using only the initial IPT phase might be compared with the full treatment. Data from the Frank et al. (1991) study showed the value of monthly maintenance IPT for patients with recurrent depression, but a series of dose-ranging studies might compare weekly, biweekly, and monthly frequency of sessions. Such studies would be comparable to phase II or III pharmacotherapy trials.

It is unclear how efficacy data for psychotherapies such as IPT will be used in health care reform—to what degree health care reform will require standardization of treatment, training credentials, and evidence of effectiveness and/or cost offset. Since clinical trials often exclude patients with complex comorbidity seen in clinical practice, reimbursement policy based on data from clinical trials should adjust for this contingency. We must learn how the efficacy of IPT in clinical research translates into effectiveness when used by general clinicians.

It is unclear whether in the future untested psychotherapies will be reimbursed or whether psychotherapy will be reimbursed at all, and, if so, with what limits on intensity and duration of treatment. Strict limits on psychotherapy reimbursement would harm many patients, including recurrent depressed patients unresponsive to medication or depressed pregnant or nursing women. The efficacy of antidepressant pharmacotherapy is unequivocal, yet medicating depressed patients without psychological management risks poor compliance and persistence of unresolved social stressors. The best interests of all psychiatric patients are ensured by access to a range of treatment modalities whose efficacy has been established in controlled clinical trials.

References

American Psychiatric Association: Diagnostic and Statistical Manual of Mental Disorders, 4th Edition. Washington, DC, American Psychiatric Association, 1994

Angus L, Gillies LA: Counselling the borderline client: an interpersonal approach. Canadian Journal of Counseling/Rev Canad Counsel 28:69–82, 1994

Barber JP, Muenz LR: The role of avoidance and obsessiveness in matching patients to cognitive and interpersonal psychotherapy: empirical findings from the Treatment for Depression Collaborative Research Program. J Consult Clin Psychol 64:951–958, 1996

Beck AT: Depression Inventory. Philadelphia, PA, Philadelphia Center for Cognitive Therapy, 1978

Blatt SJ, Quinlan DM, Pilokonis PA, et al: Impact of perfectionism and need for approval on the brief treatment of depression: the National Institute of Mental Health Treatment of Depression Collaborative Research Program revisited. J Consult Clin Psychol 63:125–132, 1995

Blom MBJ, Hoencamp E, Zwaan T: Interpersoonlijke psychotherapie voor depressie: een pilot-onderzoek. Tijdschrift voor Psychiatr 38:398–402, 1996

Brown C, Schulberg HC, Madonia MJ, et al: Treatment outcomes for primary care patients with major depression and lifetime anxiety disorders. Am J Psychiatry 153:1293–1300, 1996

Carroll KM, Rounsaville BJ, Gawin FH: A comparative trial of psychotherapies for ambulatory cocaine abusers: relapse prevention and interpersonal psychotherapy. Am J Drug Alcohol Abuse 17:229–247, 1991

Chevron ES, Rounsaville BJ: Evaluating the clinical skills of psychotherapists: a comparison of techniques. Arch Gen Psychiatry 40:1129–1132, 1983

Consumers Guide, November 1995, p 739

Depression Guideline Panel: Clinical Practice Guideline: Depression in Primary Care, Vol 1–4 (AHCPR Publ No 93-0550–0553). Rockville, MD, U.S. Department of Health and Human Services, Agency for Health Care Policy and Research, 1993

DiMascio A, Weissman MM, Prusoff BA, et al: Differential symptom reduction by drugs and psychotherapy in acute depression. Arch Gen Psychiatry 36:1450–1456, 1979

Ehlers CL, Frank E, Kupfer DJ: Social zeitgebers and biological rhythms: a unified approach to understanding the etiology of depression. Arch Gen Psychiatry 45:948–952, 1988

Elkin I, Shea MT, Watkins JT, et al: National Institute of Mental Health treatment of depression collaborative research program: general effectiveness of treatments. Arch Gen Psychiatry 46:971–982, 1989

Fairburn CG, Jones R, Peveler RC, et al: Three psychological treatments for bulimia nervosa: a comparative trial. Arch Gen Psychiatry 48:463–469, 1991

Fairburn CG, Jones R, Peveler RC, et al: Psychotherapy and bulimia nervosa: longer-term effects of interpersonal psychotherapy, behavior therapy, and cognitive behavior therapy. Arch Gen Psychiatry 50:419–428, 1993

Fairburn CG, Norman PA, Welch SL, et al: A prospective study of outcome in bulimia nervosa and the long-term effects of three psychological treatments. Arch Gen Psychiatry 52:304–312, 1995

Foley SH, Rounsaville BJ, Weissman MM, et al: Individual versus conjoint interpersonal psychotherapy for depressed patients with marital disputes. International Journal of Family Psychiatry 10:29–42, 1989

Frank E: Biological order and bipolar disorder. Paper presented at the meeting of the American Psychosomatic Society, Santa Fe, NM, March 1991a

Frank E: Interpersonal psychotherapy as a maintenance treatment for patients with recurrent depression. Psychotherapy 28:259–266, 1991b

Frank E, Kupfer DJ, Perel JM: Early recurrence in unipolar depression. Arch Gen Psychiatry 46:397–400, 1989

Frank E, Kupfer DJ, Perel JM, et al: Three-year outcomes for maintenance therapies in recurrent depression. Arch Gen Psychiatry 47:1093–1099, 1990

Frank E, Kupfer DJ, Wagner EF, et al: Efficacy of interpersonal psychotherapy as a maintenance treatment of recurrent depression. Arch Gen Psychiatry 48:1053–1059, 1991

Goldberg DP: The Detection of Psychiatric Illness by Questionnaire, Maudsley Monographs No. 21. London, England, Oxford University Press, 1972

Gurman AS, Kniskern DP: Research on marital and family therapy: progress, perspective, and prospect, in Handbook of Psychotherapy and Behavior Change. Edited by Bergin AE, Garfield SL. New York, Wiley, 1978, pp 817–902

Hamilton M: A rating scale for depression. J Neurol Neurosurg Psychiatry 25:56–62, 1960

Jarrett RB, Rush AJ: Short-term psychotherapy of depressive disorders: current status and future directions. Psychiatry 57:115–132, 1994

Karasu TB, Docherty JP, Gelenberg A, et al: Practice guideline for major depressive disorder in adults. Am J Psychiatry 150:1–26, 1993

Klein DF, Ross DC: Reanalysis of the National Institute of Mental Health Treatment of Depression Collaborative Research Program general effectiveness report. Neuropsychopharmacology 8:241–251, 1993

Klerman GL, Weissman MM: New Applications of Interpersonal Psychotherapy. Washington, DC, American Psychiatric Press, 1993

Klerman GL, DiMascio A, Weissman MM, et al: Treatment of depression by drugs and psychotherapy. Am J Psychiatry 131:186–191, 1974

Klerman GL, Weissman MM, Rounsaville BJ, et al: Interpersonal Psychotherapy of Depression. New York, Basic Books, 1984

Klerman GL, Budman S, Berwick D, et al: Efficacy of brief psychosocial intervention for symptoms of stress and distress among patients in primary care. Med Care 25:1078–1088, 1987

Klerman GL, Weissman MM, Rounsaville BJ, et al: Psicoterapia Interpersonale Della Depressione. Torino, Bollati Boringhiere, 1989

Klerman GL, Weissman MM, Markowitz JC, et al: Medication and psychotherapy, in Handbook of Psychotherapy and Behavior Change, 4th Edition. Edited by Bergin AE, Garfield SL. New York, Wiley, 1994, pp 734–782

Klerman GL, Weissman MM, Rounsaville BJ, et al: Interpersonal Psychotherapy of Depression. Translated by Hiroko Mizushima. Makoto Shimada, Yutaka Ono. Tokyo, Iwasaki Gakujyutsa, 1997

Kocsis JH, Frances AJ, Voss C, et al: Imipramine treatment for chronic depression. Arch Gen Psychiatry 45:253–257, 1988

Luborsky L: Principles of Psychoanalytic Psychotherapy: A Manual for Supportive/Expressive Treatment. New York, Basic Books, 1984

Markowitz JC: Psychotherapy of the post-dysthymic patient. Journal of Psychotherapy Practice and Research 2:157–163, 1993

Markowitz JC: Psychotherapy of dysthymia. Am J Psychiatry 151:1114–1121, 1994

Markowitz JC: Teaching interpersonal psychotherapy to psychiatric residents. Academic Psychiatry 19:167–173, 1995

Markowitz JC: Interpersonal Psychotherapy for Dysthymic Disorder. Washington, DC, American Psychiatric Press, 1997

Markowitz JC, Swartz HA: Case formulation in interpersonal psychotherapy of depression, in Handbook of Psychotherapy Case Formulation. Edited by Eels TD. New York, Guilford, 1997, pp 192–222

Markowitz JC, Klerman GL, Perry SW, et al: Interpersonal therapy of depressed HIV-seropositive patients. Hosp Community Psychiatry 43:885–890, 1992

Markowitz JC, Kocsis JH, Fishman B, et al: Treatment of HIV-positive patients with depressive symptoms. Arch Gen Psychiatry (in press)

Miller MD, Silberman RL: Using interpersonal psychotherapy with depressed elders, in A Guide to Psychotherapy and Aging: Effective Clinical Interventions in a Life-Stage Context. Edited by Zarit SH, Knight BG. Washington, DC, American Psychological Association, 1996, pp 83–99

Miller MD, Frank E, Cornes C, et al: Applying interpersonal psychotherapy to bereavement-related depression following loss of a spouse in late life. Journal of Psychotherapy Practice and Research 3:149–162, 1994

Moreau D, Mufson L, Weissman MM, et al: Interpersonal psychotherapy for adolescent depression: description of modification and preliminary application. J Am Acad Child Adolesc Psychiatry 30:642–651, 1991

Mossey JM, Knott KA, Higgins M, et al: Effectiveness of a psychosocial intervention, interpersonal counseling, for subdysthymic depression in medically ill elderly. J Gerontol A Biol Sci Med Sci 51:M172–M178, 1996

Mufson L, Fairbanks J: Interpersonal psychotherapy for depressed adolescents: a one-year naturalistic follow-up study. J Am Acad Child Adolesc Psychiatry 35:1145–1155, 1996

Mufson L, Moreau D, Weissman MM, et al (eds): Interpersonal Therapy for Depressed Adolescents. New York, Guilford, 1993

Mufson L, Moreau D, Weissman MM, et al: Modification of interpersonal psychotherapy with depressed adolescents (IPT-A): phase I and II studies. J Am Acad Child Adolesc Psychiatry 33:695–705, 1994

Müller-Popkens K, Hajak G: Interpersonelle Psychotherapie zur Behandlung von Patienten mit primärer Insomnie—Vorläufige Daten zur polysomnographischen Makroanalyse. Wien Med Wochenschr 146:303–305, 1996

Parsons T: Illness and the role of the physician: a sociological perspective. Am J Orthopsychiatry 21:452–460, 1951

Paykel ES, DiMascio A, Haskell D, et al: Effects of maintenance amitriptyline and psychotherapy on symptoms of depression. Psychol Med 5:67–77, 1975

Puig JS: Psicoterapia interpersonal, I. Rev Psiquiatría Fac Med Barna 22:91–99, 1995

Reynolds CF, Frank E, Perel JM, et al: Combined pharmacotherapy and psychotherapy in the acute and continuation treatment of elderly patients with recurrent major depression: a preliminary report. Am J Psychiatry 149:1687–1692, 1992

Reynolds CF, Frank E, Kupfer DJ, et al: Treatment outcome in recurrent major depression: a post hoc comparison of elderly ("young old") and midlife patients. Am J Psychiatry 153:1288–1292, 1996

Reynolds CF, Frank E, Houck PR, et al: Which elderly patients with

remitted depression remain well with continued interpersonal psychotherapy after discontinuation of antidepressant medication? Am
J Psychiatry 154:958–962, 1997

Rothblum ED, Sholomskas AJ, Berry C, et al: Issues in clinical trials
with the depressed elderly. J Am Geriatr Soc 30:694–699, 1982

Rounsaville BJ, Weissman MM, Prusoff BA, et al: Marital disputes and
treatment outcome in depressed women. Compr Psychiatry 20:483–
490, 1979

Rounsaville BJ, Glazer W, Wilber CH, et al: Short-term interpersonal
psychotherapy in methadone-maintained opiate addicts. Arch Gen
Psychiatry 40:629–636, 1983

Rounsaville BJ, Chevron ES, Weissman MM, et al: Training therapists
to perform interpersonal psychotherapy in clinical trials. Compr
Psychiatry 27:364–371, 1986

Rounsaville BJ, O'Malley SS, Foley SH, et al: The role of manual-guided
training in the conduct and efficacy of interpersonal psychotherapy
for depression. J Consult Clin Psychol 56:681–688, 1988

Schramm E: Interpersonelle Psychotherapie bei Depressionen und An-
deren Psychischen Störungen. Stuttgart, Schattauer, 1996

Schulberg HC, Scott CP: Depression in primary care: treating depression with interpersonal psychotherapy, in Psychotherapy in Managed Health Care: The Optimal Use of Time and Resources. Edited
by Austad CS, Berman WH. Washington, DC, American Psychological Association, 1991, pp 153–170

Schulberg HC, Scott CP, Madonia MJ, et al: Applications of interpersonal psychotherapy to depression in primary care practice, in New
Applications of Interpersonal Psychotherapy. Edited by Klerman
GL, Weissman MM. Washington, DC, American Psychiatric Press,
1993, pp 265–291

Schulberg HC, Block MR, Madonia MJ, et al: Treating major depression
in primary care practice. Arch Gen Psychiatry 53:913–919, 1996

Scott J, Ikkos G: A pilot study of interpersonal psychotherapy for the
treatment of chronic somatization in primary care. Paper presented
at the First Congress of the World Council of Psychotherapy, Vienna,
Austria, June 30–July 4, 1996

Shea MT, Elkin I, Imber SD, et al: Course of depressive symptoms over
follow-up: findings from the National Institute of Mental Health
Treatment for Depression Collaborative Research Program. Arch
Gen Psychiatry 49:782–794, 1992

Sholomskas AJ, Chevron ES, Prusoff BA, et al: Short-term interpersonal
therapy (IPT) with the depressed elderly: case reports and discussion. Am J Psychother 36:552–566, 1983

Sloane RB, Stapes FR, Schneider LS: Interpersonal therapy versus nortriptyline for depression in the elderly, in Clinical and Pharmacological Studies in Psychiatric Disorders. Edited by Burrows GD, Norman TR, Dennerstein L. London, John Libbey, 1985, pp 344–346

Sotsky SM: Pharmacotherapy and psychotherapy response in atypical depression: findings from the NIMH Treatment of Depression Collaborative Research Program. Paper presented as part of Symposium 73 at the American Psychiatric Association 150th Annual Meeting, San Diego, CA, May 1997

Sotsky SM, Glass DR, Shea MT, et al: Patient predictors of response to psychotherapy and pharmacotherapy: findings in the NIMH Treatment of Depression Collaborative Research Program. Am J Psychiatry 148:997–1008, 1991

Stuart S, Cole V: Treatment of depression following myocardial infarction with interpersonal psychotherapy. Ann Clin Psychiatry 8:203–206, 1996

Sullivan HS (ed): The Interpersonal Theory of Psychiatry. New York, WW Norton, 1953

Swartz HA, Markowitz JC, Spinelli MG: Interpersonal psychotherapy of a dysthymic, pregnant, HIV-positive woman. Journal of Psychotherapy Practice and Research 6:165–178, 1997

Thase ME, Fava M, Halbreich U, et al: A placebo-controlled, randomized clinical trial comparing sertraline and imipramine for the treatment of dysthymia. Arch Gen Psychiatry 53:777–784, 1996

Thase ME, Buysse DJ, Frank E, et al: Which depressed patients will respond to interpersonal psychotherapy? the role of abnormal EEG sleep profiles. Am J Psychiatry 154:502–509, 1997

Weissman A, Beck AT: Development and validation of the Dysfunctional Attitudes Scale: a preliminary investigation. Paper presented at the annual meeting of the American Educational Research Association, Toronto, Ontario, Canada, 1978

Weissman MM: Mastering Depression: A Patient Guide to Interpersonal Psychotherapy. Albany, NY, Graywind, 1995. Currently available through The Psychological Corporation, Order Service Center, PO Box 839954, San Antonio, TX 78283-3954, Tel 1-800-228-0752, Fax 1-800-232-1223

Weissman MM, Klerman GL, Paykel ES, et al: Treatment effects on the social adjustment of depressed patients. Arch Gen Psychiatry 30:771–778, 1974

Weissman MM, Prusoff BA, DiMascio A, et al: The efficacy of drugs and psychotherapy in the treatment of acute depressive episodes. Am J Psychiatry 136:555–558, 1979

Weissman MM, Klerman GL, Prusoff BA, et al: Depressed outpatients: results one year after treatment with drugs and/or interpersonal psychotherapy. Arch Gen Psychiatry 38:52–55, 1981

Weissman MM, Rounsaville BJ, Chevron ES: Training psychotherapists to participate in psychotherapy outcome studies: identifying and dealing with the research requirement. Am J Psychiatry 139:1442–1446, 1982

Wells KB, Stewart A, Hays RD, et al: The functioning and well-being of depressed patients: results from the medical outcomes study. JAMA 262:914–919, 1989

Wilfley DE, Agras WS, Telch CF, et al: Group cognitive-behavioral therapy and group interpersonal psychotherapy for the nonpurging bulimic individual: a controlled comparison. J Consult Clin Psychol 61:296–305, 1993

Chapter 2

Interpersonal Psychotherapy for Adolescent Depression

Laura Mufson, Ph.D., and Donna Moreau, M.D.

Interpersonal psychotherapy for depressed adolescents (IPT-A) is a brief, focused therapy modified and adapted from interpersonal psychotherapy (IPT) for depressed adults (Klerman et al. 1984). IPT traces its historical roots to the work of Harry Stack Sullivan and Adolf Meyer. Meyer (1957), drawing on Darwinian principles of biological adaptation, believed that mental illness was the result of the individual's maladaptive attempts to adjust to the social environment. Sullivan (1956) expanded on Meyer's theories and approached the understanding of psychiatric disorders from the perspective of interpersonal relationships. Klerman et al. (1984) applied the interpersonal approach to develop a short-term treatment (IPT) for the ambulatory depressed adult. They developed and published a manual with specific guidelines for conducting the therapy and created a training program for mental health professionals to be used in clinical research trials (Weissman et al. 1979). In 1995 Weissman published a patient's guide to IPT that is used in conjunction with treatment.

Although interpersonal theory recognizes the contribution that difficulties in historical interpersonal relations make to the predisposition and development of depression, the focus of IPT is on the depressive disorder's impact on the patient's current interpersonal relationships in the spheres of family, friends, and

---

Portions of this chapter have been adapted from Mufson L, Moreau D, Weissman MM: "Focus on Relationships: Interpersonal Psychotherapy for Adolescent Depression, in *Psychosocial Treatments for Child and Adolescent Disorders*. Edited by Hibbs ED, Jensen PS. Washington, DC, American Psychological Association, 1996. Used with permission.

---

co-workers (Klerman et al. 1984). Depression is conceptualized in an interpersonal context. The goals of IPT are to ameliorate the depressive symptoms and improve current interpersonal functioning in significant relationships. Personality and character change are not foci of the therapeutic process.

IPT has been tested for the treatment of adult major depression in multiple studies including three acute treatment studies (Elkin et al. 1989; Sloane et al. 1985; Weissman et al. 1974) and two maintenance trials (Frank et al. 1990; Klerman et al. 1974). IPT-A was first studied in an open clinical trial (Mufson et al. 1993), and a controlled clinical trial has just been completed.

In this chapter we focus on the rationale for the development and structure of IPT-A, the therapeutic stance of the IPT-A therapist, and the therapeutic techniques and strategies used. We review published and ongoing IPT-A research protocols and speculate on implications for future research and more widespread clinical applications.

Rationale for the Development of IPT-A

Adolescent depression is a highly prevalent disorder, with rates of depressive symptoms in epidemiological samples as high as 42% in boys and 48% in girls (Rutter et al. 1976) and rates of major depression in community- and school-based samples ranging from 0.4% to 5.7% (Chaput et al. 1997). Adolescent depression is accompanied by significant psychosocial impairment in the acute phase (Kye and Ryan 1995; Seigel et al. 1990; Strober et al. 1993) and results in persistent psychosocial impairment that extends into adulthood long after the mood component resolves (Harrington et al. 1990). Longitudinal studies have demonstrated that adolescent depression is chronic and recurrent (Garber et al. 1988; Harrington et al. 1990; Kandel and Davies 1986; Keller et al. 1988; Kovacs et al. 1984; Strober 1985; Strober et al. 1993; Welner et al. 1979) yet goes largely untreated (Keller et al. 1991), with as many as 50% of depressed adolescents not seeking or receiving clinical attention (Whitaker et al. 1990). In part, this lack of clinical attention is due to underidentification of the disorder.

Research and clinical experience also identify other barriers to treatment such as the transient nature of some adolescent depressions (Garber et al. 1988; Harrington et al. 1990; Keller et al. 1988), the adolescent's resistance to treatment, and the parental resistance to identifying a child as in need of psychiatric services.

Numerous clinical reports and articles in the psychiatric literature concentrate on psychotherapy with depressed adolescents. However, there are few published reports (Brent et al. 1997; Lewinsohn et al. 1990; Reynolds and Imber 1988; Robbins et al. 1989; Wilkes et al. 1994) of well-designed scientific studies that demonstrate the efficacy of any one treatment. Pharmacological treatment has received (and continues to receive) a great deal of scientific and clinical attention, but the results so far are discouraging: In the majority of studies, antidepressant medication does not appear to be superior to placebo (Chaput et al. 1997; Kramer and Feiguine 1981; Ryan et al. 1986). The study by Emslie et al. (in press) is the first to report a significant effect for medication (fluoxetine) over placebo in the treatment of depressed children and adolescents. As the methodology and design of these studies are applied to larger numbers of adolescents, we may be able to determine which antidepressants work for which patients. Even so, the acute and chronic psychosocial impairment that accompanies adolescent depression argues strongly for the use of a psychotherapeutic intervention, either alone or eventually in conjunction with medication.

Normal developmental processes and the accompanying tasks that occur as the adolescent matures present expected barriers to the adolescent's engaging in psychotherapy (McCarthy 1989; Swift and Wonderlich 1990). Cognitive development measured by concentration, capacity for introspection, and the shift to formal operations varies by age, intelligence, adjustment, and individuality and may limit the adolescent's potential to engage in a therapeutic working alliance (McCarthy 1989). Adolescents struggle with issues of separation and individuation from their parents and the accompanying feelings of ambivalence about the struggle. This situation explains the adolescent's preference for action over thought and verbal communications. A precarious sense of self-esteem contributes to externalization and avoidance of introspection (Swift and Wonderlich 1990). Many depressed adolescents are not only resistant to seeking treatment but also frequently miss multiple appointments and conclude therapy early. They often flounder in open-ended psychotherapy, not knowing what to talk about or how to focus their sessions. In addition, if the depressive symptoms are of a transient nature, there is little impetus to continue in treatment. IPT-A addresses these developmentally based barriers to treatment by offering a time-limited therapy (12 weeks), a clear explanation of what the adolescent can expect from the therapy, active involvement on the part of the therapist, and structured sessions with a mutually agreed upon focus. In addition, IPT-A by definition focuses on the interpersonal issues that constitute the core of the adolescent's experience and developmental tasks.

IPT-A draws on prior experience in the field of brief psychotherapy in determining which adolescents are suitable patients (Klerman et al. 1984; Reich and Neenan 1986; Sifneos 1981). The adolescent must be motivated and willing to engage in the therapeutic work. Expectations for the therapy must be realistic. It is important that the adolescent have a history of functioning effectively in one or more areas of life. In addition, IPT-A stipulates that the patient not be psychotic, actively suicidal, or using alcohol or drugs. The patient must have parental support for the therapy and be of normal intelligence.

Description of IPT-A

The modifications of IPT for depressed adolescents (IPT-A) address issues that present themselves in adolescent treatment cases, using the IPT framework. The overall goals and problem areas of IPT (grief, interpersonal role disputes, role transitions, and interpersonal deficits) are identical in IPT-A. A fifth problem area, the single-parent family, has been added because of its frequent occurrence, its association with depression, and the conflicts it engenders for adolescents. The treatment has been adapted to address developmental issues most common to adolescents, including separation from parents, exploration of authority in relation to parents, development of dyadic interpersonal relationships with members of the opposite sex, initial experience with death of a relative or friend, and peer pressures. Strategies were developed for including family members in various phases of the treatment as needed and for addressing special issues that arise in the treatment of adolescents such as school refusal, physical or sexual abuse, suicidality, aggression, and involvement of a child protective service agency. All of the modifications have been organized into a treatment manual designed specifically for depressed adolescents (Mufson et al. 1993).

Specific Treatment Techniques

IPT-A is designed as a once-weekly, 12-week treatment. If a crisis develops, the therapist and patient may meet for one or two additional sessions in the same week to help see the patient through the crisis. The goals of the treatment are to reduce depressive symptoms and address the interpersonal problems associated with the onset of the depression. The two main approaches for achieving these goals are to identify one or two problem areas as the focus of treatment and to emphasize the interpersonal nature of the problem or problems as they occur in current relationships. The treatment is divided into three phases: 1) the initial phase, 2) the middle phase, and 3) the termination phase.

Initial Phase

The initial phase, sessions one through four, identifies the depressive symptoms and the relevant problem areas and establishes the treatment contract. The six tasks that need to be accomplished include 1) conducting a diagnostic assessment that includes reviewing the symptoms with the patient, giving the syndrome a name, explaining depression and its treatment, giving the patient the sick role, and evaluating the need for medication; 2) assessing the type and nature of the patient's social and familial relationships (the interpersonal inventory) and relating the depression to the interpersonal context; 3) identifying the problem area(s); 4) explaining the rationale and intent of the treatment; 5) setting a treatment contract with the patient; and 6) explaining the patient's expected role in the treatment.

The therapist reviews current and past interpersonal relationships as they relate to current depressive symptoms. He or she also clarifies the nature of the interactions with significant others, expectations of the adolescent and significant others for the relationships, the satisfying and unsatisfying aspects of the relationships, and the patient's desired changes in the relationships.

Frequency and Timing of Sessions

The telephone is used with adolescents to maintain contact and ensure greater flexibility in the timing and spacing of sessions. During the first 4 weeks of treatment, the therapist may check in with the adolescent, or vice versa, by telephone once a week to provide additional support for engagement in the therapeutic process. These contacts may help to establish trust between the therapist and the adolescent in that the adolescent can perceive the therapist as being concerned and involved. Similarly, the adolescent is encouraged to call if the need arises. If a patient is unable to attend a session because of a school or family obligation and rescheduling is impossible, the therapist conducts an abbreviated session on the telephone to prevent disruption in the therapeutic work. Telephone contact as a substitute for sessions is responsive to the adolescent's increased need to resume normal activities with recovery and to the real-life obligations of some adolescents.

Involving the School

Maintaining an alliance with the school system is important for the therapist. He or she should obtain the adolescent's and parents' consent to contact the school in the initial session of treatment. The therapist and school may find it necessary to work out an individual academic program to reintegrate the school-avoidant adolescent back into school and to assess the effectiveness of the therapeutic intervention. The therapist can assume the patient-advocate role with the educational system, educating teachers about the effects of a depressive episode on school functioning. He or she should generally maintain contact with the school, obtaining information from school personnel on the patient's behavior, social relationships, and academic performance to better inform the treatment regarding the most pressing problems or evidence of improvement. Similarly, the school should be made to feel that officials can call the therapist with any questions regarding behavioral observations of the patient. It is very important to know how the patient is functioning in one of his or her major roles so that the therapist can monitor the effectiveness of the interventions.

Involving the Parents

The therapist must also maintain an alliance with the parents when treating adolescents. It is important for the therapist to help the parents take the patient's problem seriously and to adjust to the notion of having an adolescent who is depressed, in addition to helping them accept any role they may be playing in the adolescent's difficulties. If there is a hostile dispute between the adolescent and parent(s), or the adolescent has been coerced into coming for treatment, the therapist should help the adolescent and the parent(s) see that the treatment is an effort to resolve the dispute in a time-limited therapy. This approach may alleviate the tension and increase compliance with treatment. Parents may also be directly involved in the therapy sessions with the adolescent, depending on the nature of the interpersonal problem (this issue is further discussed under the appropriate problem area). The parents are requested to attend an initial introduction session and summary termination session to discuss the implications of the treatment on the adolescent and his or her family. Participation in the middle phase occurs as needed.

The Sick Role

The adolescent is encouraged to think of him- or herself as in treatment and is given a limited sick role: The adolescent is

---

viewed as having an illness but is not excused from performing his or her normal duties, such as attending school. Despite the tendency to withdraw socially or avoid usual social expectations when depressed, the adolescent is encouraged to maintain his or her usual social roles in the family, at school, and with friends. The therapist advises the parents to be supportive and to encourage the adolescent to engage in as many normal activities as possible while understanding that the quality of the performance may not be as good as before the onset of depression. Patient and parents are advised that the quality of the work will probably improve as the depression remits. Together, the assignment of the sick role and psychoeducation can help to reverse negative behaviors by family members.

Treatment Contract

At the end of the initial phase, the therapist and patient together make an explicit treatment contract. The contract specifies which of the five problem areas will be the focus of the treatment, as well as confidentiality, the frequency of sessions, rules regarding missed appointments, level of parental involvement in treatment, and patient's role in the treatment. When specifying the problem area, it is imperative that the therapist determine whether the adolescent agrees with the formulation. Having the adolescent explain the formulation in his or her own words to ensure that it is understood correctly is important. The adolescent is told that further treatment can and will be arranged if necessary at the end of the 12 weeks. The middle phase can begin once an agreement has been reached on the treatment plan.

Middle Phase

During the middle phase, sessions five through eight, the therapist and patient begin to work directly on one or two of the designated problem areas. The goals of the middle phase are to alleviate the symptoms, clarify the problem, identify effective strategies to attack the problem, implement the interventions, and improve interpersonal functioning. The therapist encourages the patient to discuss feelings, monitors the depressive symptoms, and continues to work with the family to support the treatment. Techniques, which vary depending on the problem area being addressed, include the following: exploratory questioning, encouragement of affect, linkage of affect with events, clarification of conflicts, communication analysis, and behavior change techniques such as role-playing. The therapist offers continuous feedback about the use of strategies and observed changes in the patient's functioning in an effort to improve the patient's self-esteem.

Therapist and patient work as a team. Together they assess the accuracy of the initial formulation of the problem area and shift the focus of the treatment to events occurring outside of the session that appear related to the patient's depressive symptomatology. Interpersonal style in the session is discussed as it relates to interactions that may be occurring outside of the session. The middle phase also may involve other family members as needed to address situations both inside and outside of the sessions. Education about depression and interpersonal relationships continues.

Problem Areas

Grief. Grief is a problem only if it is prolonged or becomes abnormal; IPT-A has been used to treat abnormal grief. There are three types of pathological mourning (distorted grief, delayed grief, or chronic grief) that can lead to depression either immediately following the loss or at some later time when the patient is reminded of the loss (Raphael 1983). Loss of a parent during adolescence necessitates premature separation and individuation in addition to the usual tasks of mourning. Common reactions include withdrawal and depressed feelings, a display of pseudomaturity, overidentification with the deceased, and regression to earlier developmental stages (Krupnick 1984). The adolescent also may experience feelings of abandonment. Rather than appearing as affective symptoms, the difficulties may manifest themselves in behavioral problems such as drug or alcohol abuse, sexual promiscuity, or truancy (Raphael 1983).

The role of IPT-A in the treatment of normal grief reactions in adolescents is to assist the adolescent in separating from the deceased by helping him or her accept the actual loss of and dependency on the deceased (Raphael 1983). Facilitating the work of a normal grief reaction may prevent a future abnormal reaction. Although there is no systematic evidence to support this belief, several adolescents with normal grief reactions have been treated and have improved with treatment. Long-term follow-up studies to demonstrate prophylaxis have not been conducted.

IPT-A similarly addresses the depression associated with pathological grief reactions. The therapist helps the patient discuss the loss and identify and experience the associated feelings. As the patient begins to grieve appropriately and the symptoms dissipate, the loss should be better understood and accepted and the patient freed to pursue new relationships. One must consider the adolescent's role in the family system, the nature of the relationship lost, the remaining social support network, and the adolescent's psychological maturity in addressing the impact of the loss.

The Case of *A*

A, a 13-year-old adolescent male, presented for treatment because of increasing problems in school and at home since his younger sister's death in a traffic accident a few months previously. *A* described a decrease in concentration in school, an inability to make decisions, increased irritability and behavior problems at home with his younger brother, feelings of guilt over his relationship with his deceased sister, increased tearfulness, feelings of wanting to be dead so that he could be with his sister, and loss of interest in usual activities. He met criteria for uncomplicated bereavement.

A reported many guilty feelings about how he should have conducted his relationship with his sister (e.g., spent more time with her, taken her more places, and not teased her as much). He was very worried about the grief his mother was experiencing and did not want to upset her by telling her about his own feelings. He expressed the wish that it had been he who had died because his mother had another son but not another daughter.

A felt a lack of control over his life and generalized this feeling to his academic performance; he no longer felt that his effort affected the results on his tests and thus decreased his efforts at school. Because of his inability to talk with anyone about his feelings, *A* grew increasingly irritable, particularly with his younger brother, whom *A* felt was getting more attention because he had been at the scene of the accident.

The therapist's first intervention was to have *A* discuss his feelings about his sister, their relationship, and the accident in an attempt to correct his misconceptions about his responsibility for what had happened. In addition, the therapist talked with *A* about his feelings of being unloved by his mother, being treated differently from his brother, and insecurity about his place in the family. *A*'s mother was already in treatment to deal with her own grief over the accident. Subsequent sessions focused on how *A*'s feeling about life in general had changed since the accident and how they might be affecting things such as his school performance and his relationship with his brother. *A*, with the help of his therapist, explored his feelings of guilt, loss, abandonment, anger, and fear about something else happening to the family. Through expression of these feelings, *A* experienced some relief from the anger and guilty feelings and improved his ability to talk about what he was feeling rather than acting it out through disruptive behavior at home and at school. *A* felt a decreased need to punish himself for his sister's death and made a concerted effort to improve his schoolwork, with much success. He became more involved in extracurricular activities and improved the quality of his friendships.

Interpersonal role disputes.   An interpersonal dispute is defined as a situation in which the individual and at least one significant other person have nonreciprocal expectations about their relationship. Adolescents' role disputes commonly occur with parents over issues of sexuality, authority, money, and life values (Miller 1974). Often these conflicting values lead to different expectations for the adolescent's behavior. This conflict also can be seen frequently in the normal adolescent rebellion against parental authority.

The general strategies for treating interpersonal disputes are essentially the same for adolescents as they are for adults: identify the dispute, make choices about negotiations, reassess expectations for the relationship, clarify role changes, and modify communication patterns for resolution of the dispute. What differs in treating adolescents' role disputes is the nature of the problems and the involvement of the parents. The therapist needs to explain to the adolescent and the parents how the interpersonal role dispute contributes to depressive symptoms and how resolution of the dispute can alleviate the symptoms. It can be useful to involve the parent(s) with whom there is a dispute and to facilitate the negotiation of the relationship in the session with the therapist. Improvements may take the form of a change in the expectations and behavior of the patient, the other person, or both. The goal of IPT-A is to help the adolescent clarify his or her expectations for the relationship, evaluate which expectations are realistic, and find strategies for coping with the immutable expectations.

Role transitions. Role transitions are defined as the changes that occur as a result of progression from one social role to another. A person can experience depression when he or she has difficulty coping with life changes associated with a role change or if significant others (i.e., parents) have difficulty adjusting to the role change. The transition may result in impaired social functioning if it occurs too rapidly or is experienced as a loss by the individual. Normal role transitions for adolescents include 1) passage into puberty, 2) shift from group to dyadic relationships, 3) initiation of sexual relationships or desires, 4) separation from parents and family, and 5) work, college, or career planning. Problems arise when parents are unable to accept the transition or when the adolescent is unable to cope with the changes. Role transitions also can be thrust on adolescents as a result of unanticipated circumstances. Unforeseen or imposed role transitions include parenthood or a change in family role caused by divorce, remarriage, death, illness, impairment in parent, or separation from parent. Problems that occur with expected and unexpected role transitions include loss of self-esteem, failure to meet one's own and others' expectations, increasing pressures and responsibilities, and inability to separate from family or family's inability to allow that separation (Erikson 1968).

Adolescents' ability to cope with unforeseen circumstances rests on prior psychological functioning and social supports. Role transitions can be perceived as a loss to the adolescent, particularly if he or she felt more competent in the old role and is uncertain about his or her ability to fill the new role. Consequently, the psychological reaction to the transition can resemble that of mourning.

If the role transition problem involves changes in family roles, the therapist may include the parents in several sessions to help support the adolescent or, if necessary, help the family members adjust to the normative role transition so that they do not restrict the adolescent's development and impair his or her functioning. If family members are adjusting more easily to the transition, they will hopefully facilitate an easier transition for the adolescent.

The Case of B

B, a 16-year-old adolescent female, lived with her mother and two siblings. Although her parents had never lived together, her father lived nearby and she enjoyed a good relationship with him. B presented to the outpatient depression clinic with symptoms of sad mood, increased irritability, social withdrawal, decreased concentration, decreased grades, loss of interest in friends, loss of appetite, early and middle insomnia, increased heart rate, and tingling in hands periodically when at home. Her symptoms had been present for approximately 2 months and had been precipitated by a breakup with a boyfriend that resulted in conflict with her mother. She met DSM-III-R (American Psychiatric Association 1987) criteria for major depression.

B described her parents, particularly her mother, as very old-fashioned in regard to dating. B had brought home a boyfriend but had decided that she did not like him and ended the relationship. Her mother became angry about the way she conducted her social life, felt she was spending too much time with boys, and increased restrictions on her social life. While her mother was away for 2 weeks, B met and began to date another boy. She was too afraid to discuss her new relationship, and her concealment of the relationship increased her anxiety and feelings of depression.

The identified problem area was role transitions. The therapist focused on the patient's transition from a young girl to an adolescent who was beginning to date. Discussion focused on the patient examining her mother's concerns, understanding her own expectations for dating, and learning to communicate with her mother about her need for increasing independence while still remaining under her guidance and supervision. The therapist and B frequently role-played how she might tell her mother about her new boyfriend, elicit her mother's concerns, and discuss them rationally so that they could work out a mutually agreeable plan. Although her mother was unable to attend sessions, B was able to communicate to her about her desire for a relationship. B told her mother that she felt the relationship should not preclude her from remaining a part of the family as her daughter. She expressed her views on dating and worked out a compromise that was acceptable to her mother and herself. As her communication with her mother improved, the conflict and anxiety decreased and her concentration, mood, and grades improved.

Interpersonal deficits.   Interpersonal deficits are identified when an individual appears to lack the requisite social skills to establish and maintain appropriate relationships within and outside of the family. Interpersonal deficits can impede the adolescent's achievement of developmental tasks. These tasks are primarily social and include making same-age friends, participating in extracurricular activities, becoming part of a peer group, beginning to date, and learning to make choices regarding exclusive relationships, career, and sexuality (Hersen and Van Hasselt 1987). As a result of interpersonal deficits, the adolescent may be socially isolated from peer groups and relationships, which can lead to feelings of depression and inadequacy. These feelings of depression can in turn lead to increased social withdrawal and result in a lag in interpersonal skills when the depression resolves.

The focus of treatment is on interpersonal deficits that are more a consequence of the depression than personality traits that result in isolation. The strategies for treating adolescents include reviewing past significant relationships and exploring repetitive or parallel interpersonal problems. New strategies for approaching situations are identified and discussed. The patient is encouraged to apply these strategies to current issues. The therapist may utilize role-playing of problematic interpersonal situations and discussion of patient-therapist interactions, enabling the adolescent to explore and practice new communication skills and interpersonal behaviors and engendering a sense of social competence in the adolescent that can generalize to other situations.

Single-parent families.   Single-parent homes arise for a variety of reasons. Each situation presents unique emotional conflicts for the adolescent and the custodial parent. Depending on the circumstances, children of single-parent families can function without significant problems or can experience a myriad of problems, including depression. The intensity of the depressive reaction is likely to be related to the degree of separation, its abruptness, and whether it has happened before (Jacobson and Jacobson 1987). The child's relationship with the absent parent is affected, and the relationship with the remaining parent is also frequently altered.

IPT-A identifies several tasks for the treatment of the affected adolescent: 1) acknowledging that the departure of a parent is a significant disruption in his or her life; 2) addressing feelings of loss, rejection, abandonment, and/or punishment by the departed parent; 3) clarifying remaining expectations for his or her relationship with the absent parent; 4) negotiating a working relationship with the remaining parent; 5) establishing a relationship with the removed parent, if possible; and 6) accepting the permanence of the current situation. In discussing the feelings associated with the parent's departure, it can be helpful to have the custodial or noncustodial parent, or both, participate in a session. The focus of the session is to discuss the parent's recollection of the spouse and to correct any misconceptions the adolescent may have about the parents' relationship. It also may be helpful to have a session with a parent alone, specifically to discuss parenting issues of adolescents, including appropriate discipline and restrictions on their behavior.

The Case of C

C was a 14-year-old adolescent girl living alone with her mother. Her parents had been divorced since she was very young. Her father lived nearby and visited regularly. C presented with decreased concentration and poor school performance, increased irritability and crying, headaches, depressed mood, suicidal ideation, social withdrawal, loss of appetite, early and middle insomnia, and panic attacks.

At the time she presented to the outpatient clinic, she and her mother were sharing a room in her grandmother's apartment because of financial troubles. C was experiencing increased conflict with both her mother and grandmother. She felt as though she never had any quiet place to herself. During this time she continued her contact with her father and told him about the stress of so many people living in a small space. In the fourth week of treatment, she and her mother moved to their own apartment, but C was very worried about how they could afford it and what that pressure was going to do to her mother. She felt guilty about complaining to her mother. She also expressed much anger at her father because he always wanted to come over and joke around with her but had not been making his child support payments or giving her an allowance, as had been mandated by the courts. She felt the need to stand up for her mother and to convince him to make the payments; he responded by telling her that she favored her mother over him. C felt very trapped in her relationship with her father and guilty that she had angry feelings toward him.

The therapist identified her problem area as related to living in a single-parent family with a father who did not provide for her financially and emotionally but still demanded allegiance to him over the mother. C's father refused to participate in the treatment, and C wanted to pull away from her relationship with him because of the conflicting feelings she had toward him. The therapist focused on discussing and clarifying C's expectations for her relationship with her father and what she perceived were her mother's expectations for her own relationship with her ex-husband. Her mother participated in these sessions to help clarify for her daughter her own feelings about her ex-husband and what type of relationship she wished for C to have with him and to relieve C of the need to defend her mother's needs to her father. These discussions led C to realize that she was not responsible for her father's behavior or for the resolution of the problems between her parents. Different ways of communicating her feelings to her parents were explored. C was able to delineate more realistic expectations for her relationship with her father and to resume her visits with him with these new terms in mind. With increased clarification of the issues between her and her parents, and improved communication and negotiation of her place in regard to her parents' custody arrangement, C's depression and anxiety symptoms resolved.

Termination Phase

The termination phase lasts approximately from sessions nine through twelve. Termination is addressed at the beginning of treatment and should be discussed periodically during the course of therapy. The adolescent's two main tasks of termination are 1) to give up the relationship with the therapist and 2) to establish a sense of competence to deal with future problems. Many patients are unaware of having any feelings about the end of treatment; others may hesitate to acknowledge that they have come to value the relationship with the therapist. Patients and families should be advised that a slight recurrence of symptoms as termination approaches is common; it is not unusual for patients to have feelings of apprehension, anger, or sadness, but the appearance of such feelings does not necessarily portend a relapse. To support the patient's ability to cope with problems, the therapist should highlight the patient's skills and external supports.

The IPT-A therapist conducts a final termination session with the adolescent alone and then with the family members who have been involved in the treatment, usually a parent or parents. The sessions conducted during this phase should include an explicit discussion of feelings engendered by the end of treatment, a review of strategies learned and goals accomplished, recognition of the adolescent's areas of competence, and goal-directed anticipation of possible future episodes. Termination with family members addresses the same issues. In addition, the therapist and family discuss any changes that occurred in the family as a result of the treatment. The therapist should assist family members in anticipating the possibility of future episodes of depression and educate them as to possible warning signs of recurrence and appropriate management of recurrent episodes.

Occasions may arise in which therapist and adolescent together decide that further treatment is needed. This decision can be made for several reasons: 1) the depression has not fully remitted, 2) the adolescent may now be able to work on other issues since the depression has remitted, or 3) the therapy is serving as a stabilizing force in an otherwise chaotic environment. If uncertainty exists about whether to continue in another type of treatment, the therapist should advise the adolescent to take a few weeks without treatment and then call the therapist to reassess the need for further treatment. If it is clear at termination that the adolescent needs further treatment, an appropriate referral should be arranged. Long-term treatment may be indicated for patients with long-standing interpersonal problems or chronic or recurrent depression.

Special Issues

The therapist often encounters special issues in his or her work with adolescents, including indications for medication, nonnuclear families, the suicidal patient, the assaultive patient, school refusal, substance abuse, notification of protective service agencies in cases of physical or sexual abuse, learning disabilities, and adolescents with sexual identity problems. Although the techniques for treating these issues are not unique to IPT-A, they are placed within the interpersonal treatment contract and framework, which is discussed in the following sections.

Antidepressant Medication in Conjunction With IPT-A

The decision to use antidepressant medication in depressed adolescents is a clinical and medical one made by a child-adolescent psychiatrist in collaboration with the treating clinician if that clinician is not a psychiatrist. Antidepressant medication is not contraindicated during IPT-A; in fact, it may be a useful adjunct treatment for severely depressed adolescents whose symptoms do not remit during the initial stages of treatment. Adolescents who are treated on an outpatient basis are rarely started on antidepressant medication before the fourth week of treatment. Information regarding their depression, based on self-report and clinician-rated scales, is systematically reviewed every 4 weeks or more often if the treating clinician thinks it necessary to do so. If by the fourth week of treatment the adolescent is still significantly depressed based on these reports, then antidepressant medication is recommended as an adjunctive treatment. Indications for medication by the fourth week include persistent depressed mood, insomnia, poor concentration, school refusal, social isolation, hopelessness, and persistent thoughts of death.

The decision to use medication is discussed in a joint session with the psychiatrist, therapist, patient, and parents. Prescriptions are given to the parents or to another responsible adult, who will then be instructed on appropriate administration of the medication. If there are two treating therapists (one for medication and one for counseling), a plan of weekly communication throughout the course of dual treatment should be agreed on to keep each other abreast of changes in mental status, compliance with each aspect of the treatment, and any reported side effects of the medication. The adolescent and parent should be informed about what role each therapist plays in the treatment. Appointments should be coordinated to maximize the adolescent's participation in both aspects of the treatment.

Nonnuclear Families

For various reasons, some adolescents live in alternate arrangements (i.e., *nonnuclear families*), including the homes of other relatives, foster homes, and group homes. Reasons for these alternate arrangements include death, abandonment, intervention by protective service agencies, irreconcilable differences, and illness. The therapist's task with these adolescents is to engage the relative, foster family, or leader from the group home as he or she would engage the parents. As with the parents, these persons are important in the adolescent's daily life and must be educated about the nature of depression and the ways to support the adolescent in his or her recovery and, if necessary, participate in the treatment to facilitate changes in the home environment that will play a role in the adolescent's recovery.

Suicidal Patient

Although completed suicide in adolescence is rare, suicide attempts and suicidal ideation are highly prevalent (Shaffer et al. 1988). Evaluation for suicidality is a critical part of the initial evaluation, and suicidality should be monitored throughout the treatment. The adolescent should be asked if he or she has thought about death, about wanting to die, and about killing him- or herself. The therapist should be very specific in his or her questioning and obtain specific answers. He or she should also assess the intention and lethality of the patient's past suicide attempts, current suicidal ideation, and future plans. Based on this assessment, and taking into account the stability of the home and family, the therapist must determine whether the adolescent is an acute suicide risk. If the therapist is uncertain, a second opinion should be sought. Any adolescent who is an acute suicide risk is not a candidate for IPT-A and usually requires psychiatric hospitalization.

The suitability of an adolescent with suicidal ideation for IPT-A depends on his or her capacity to establish and maintain a therapeutic alliance with the therapist. The cornerstone of this alliance is the adolescent's assurance that he or she will not make a suicide attempt and will notify the therapist or go to an emergency room immediately if the urge becomes compelling. The task of the therapist is not only to monitor the adolescent's suicidality but also to address the inappropriate use of suicide as a means of communicating feelings of anger or distress or as a means of resolving a conflict.

Assaultive Patient

Although the frequency of treating a homicidal adolescent patient is low, some adolescents may express feelings of aggression and/or report violent behavior on occasion. Patients should be assessed for thoughts of hurting other persons in conjunction with the evaluation of suicidal behavior. As in the assessment of suicide, it is very important for the therapist to ask highly specific questions about the intent and the feasibility of going through with the action. Based on this assessment, the therapist must determine whether the adolescent is at risk for harming another person. If so, the therapist (by law in some but not all states) must hospitalize the patient and has a duty to warn the intended victim of the patient's wishes.

An adolescent who is a serious risk for homicidal behavior is not a candidate for IPT-A. One who expresses anger and hostility in vague threats to others may be a candidate for IPT-A if he or she is able to establish a therapeutic alliance with the therapist, feel able to control his or her behavior, and feel capable of making an agreement with the therapist that the threats will not be acted on while in treatment. As part of the IPT-A treatment, the therapist educates the adolescent about more appropriate methods of communicating anger or upset feelings and ways to diffuse his or her anger.

School Refusal

As a result of feelings of fatigue, poor concentration, and anhedonia, some depressed adolescents are unable to attend school regularly. Moreover, when they have been out of school for a week or two, they may conclude that they are too far behind to catch up and are embarrassed to go back to school after their absence. Consequently, they remain home for an extended period. It is important that the therapist question the adolescent and parents about school attendance during the initial evaluation. The therapist's role should be to stress the importance of returning to school and to enlist the assistance of the parents and school in ensuring the adolescent's rapid return. The therapist should explain to the adolescent that although he or she may not feel like going back and may be embarrassed, the embarrassment will dissipate after the first day and he or she will feel better by being productive in school. The adolescent should be told that his or her concentration will improve as the depression resolves. Throughout the treatment, the therapist should continue to check on the adolescent's school attendance and performance and be in contact with the school as necessary.

Substance Abuse by the Adolescent

Part of the screening and history of an adolescent should include a complete history of drug and alcohol use or abuse. Other family members should be interviewed about the adolescent's drug use, even though they may be ignorant of such abuse. If necessary, the adolescent should be referred for drug treatment before IPT-A is started. To participate in IPT-A, the adolescent must not be abusing or using any substances and must make a commitment to maintain a drug-free life. If the therapist feels that the drug use is a primary problem and the depression is secondary to the drug abuse, the adolescent should be referred to a drug treatment center. The therapist can help the adolescent deal with peer pressure and family dynamics that lead to drug use and engage another family member who may be an additional source of support in the patient's abstinence from drugs.

Protective Service Agencies

Protective service agencies are designed to protect the welfare of children when their environments are harmful or neglectful. Each state has its own agency for accepting and dealing with reports and its own laws governing when and how to report a case. A child may already be in the jurisdiction of a protective service agency when he or she begins therapy, or it may be the duty of the therapist to report the child to the protective service agency if information about possible harm to the child is uncovered in the course of treatment. The therapist contacting a protective service agency can disrupt the therapeutic alliance with the child or parent; he or she must be alert to this possibility and work with the adolescent and parent to help them understand that the service was notified to alleviate a stressful situation for both child and parent and to provide help. The therapist should emphasize that the protective service agency is a means to provide the adolescent with increased social support so that the family can function more effectively.

Sexual Abuse

As with all of the special issues, the therapist should carefully evaluate the adolescent for any past or current history of sexual abuse. Frequent symptoms that might indicate a past history of abuse include depression, suicide, sexual promiscuity, severe anxiety about sex, and conduct problems (Browne and Finkelhor 1986). Evaluating for substance abuse requires sensitivity and time. The adolescent may not reveal the abuse during the initial visits but rather during the course of treatment as he or she begins to trust the therapist. If the abuse is ongoing, the therapist is required by law to contact a protective service agency for children so that the agency can intervene with the family and provide the appropriate social services to the family or adolescent. If the abuse is current, the adolescent may not be appropriate for treatment with IPT-A, because IPT-A is not designed to deal with the acute or long-term consequences of sexual abuse. If the abuse was in the past, the therapist still needs a detailed history of the interpersonal context in which the abuse occurred so that an accurate picture of the familial relationship can be ascertained.

Learning Disabilities

Depression is commonly associated with cognitive impairments during its acute stages. A psychosocial history helps the therapist to distinguish between long-standing learning disabilities and impairments secondary to the depressive episode. This task is made more difficult when the patient has long-standing depressive symptoms or a personality style that presents with what appear to be cognitive limitations. Psychological or educational testing can be useful in identifying learning disabilities. When learning disabilities are diagnosed, special educational resources are necessary and the therapist needs to arrange to meet this need in conjunction with the school system. Cognitive impairments secondary to the depression resolve when the depressive symptoms resolve. The child and parents should be made aware of the etiology of the child's impairment and revise their expectations accordingly. Severe expressive and receptive language disabilities preclude treatment with IPT-A.

Adolescents With Sexual Identity Problems

Adolescence is the time when people begin to form intimate dyadic relationships, usually with partners of the opposite sex and for some adolescents with partners of the same sex. Exploration of sexual relationships with different partners is common. Adolescents who find that their sexual interest is exclusively with partners of the same sex can feel isolated and alone. Those who feel attracted to both same- and opposite-sex partners may feel confused about their sexual orientation. The role of the therapist is to help adolescents explore their sexual feelings and concerns about their orientation in a nonjudgmental context. In addition, it may be appropriate to identify the association between an adolescent's state of confusion and his or her depression. It is also possible that the adolescent is comfortable with and has accepted his or her sexual orientation; in such a situation, the therapist must be supportive of the decision. It is important for the therapist to keep these discussions confidential unless the adolescent has a desire to share the information with others.

Research on IPT-A

Dr. Laura Mufson directs the IPT-A research program at the New York State Psychiatric Institute. She has developed a detailed therapist training program that has been used in her research studies and has conducted pilot efficacy studies of IPT-A to determine treatment efficacy. Two studies have been conducted: a preliminary open clinical trial of IPT-A and a controlled clinical trial with random assignment. This section includes a discussion of the procedures and outcomes of both studies.

Therapist Training

In preparation for conducting the open clinical trial, Mufson was trained as an IPT therapist, created videotapes of IPT-A to train other therapists, and tested a battery of outcome assessments in depressed adolescents. Her training in IPT was conducted in accordance with the methods used in the National Institute of Mental Health (NIMH) Treatment of Depression Collaborative Research Program (Elkin et al. 1989; Weissman et al. 1982). The IPT manual was modified and adapted for use with adolescents, and a clinic was identified within which to conduct the study. These procedures are the model for the IPT-A training program being used in the controlled clinical trial.

Open Clinical Trial

The purpose of the open clinical trial was similar to that of a phase II psychopharmacology trial. The goal was to gain experience with the therapy, look at dose response, and assess the feasibility of using IPT-A with an adolescent population. The sample was composed of 14 depressed adolescents between the ages of 12 and 18 years who were referred for treatment to the Babies Hospital–Child Anxiety and Depression Clinic or who responded to an advertisement to participate in a research project on treatment for adolescent depression sponsored by the Department of Child Psychiatry Clinical Research Center (see Mufson et al. 1994 for a complete description of the open trial procedures).

Outcome

The mean age of the patients was 15.4 years. The patients attended an average of 10 therapy sessions in 12 weeks. In general, the results indicated a significant decrease in adolescents' depressive symptomatology and symptoms of psychological and physical distress, as well as a significant improvement in functioning over the course of treatment. At the end of the protocol, none of the patients met DSM-III-R criteria for any depressive disorder (Mufson et al. 1994).

One-Year Naturalistic Follow-Up

Of the 14 patients available from the open clinical trial, 10 participated in a 1-year naturalistic follow-up study (Mufson et al. 1994). Of the four patients who did not participate, one was in college, one did not live near the study site but was not depressed by the mother's phone report, one refused, and one was living in a runaway shelter. No significant differences were found between those who did and did not participate on demographics or clinical characteristics at baseline. None of the boys participated in the follow-up study. The follow-up assessment was identical to the measures collected during the open clinical trial, with the addition of a life events questionnaire. The mean age of the girls was 17.5 years. At follow-up, only one patient met DSM-III-R criteria for major depression and dysthymic disorder. This patient, however, had withdrawn from the open clinical trial at week 4 and, in addition, had a significant childhood history of sexual abuse. The remaining patients reported few depressive symptoms and good social functioning despite a substantial number of adverse life events during the intervening year. All were attending school regularly, and there were no reports of suicides, hospitalizations, or pregnancies. The findings of Mufson and Fairbanks (1996) suggest that the majority of adolescents maintained their state of recovery from depression up until 1 year after completing treatment with IPT-A.

Limitations

Although the results of the open trial were encouraging for the use of IPT-A in the treatment of depressed adolescents, the results need to be viewed in light of their limitations. All of the IPT-A treatment had been conducted by one therapist, who developed the treatment; therefore, it was unclear whether the patients' improvement was due to the therapist or the techniques of the treatment. To address this issue, treatment in the controlled clinical trial was conducted by three other therapists who were trained in IPT-A. Secondly, because of the small sample size and lack of control group, the investigator did not know how many of the patients would have gotten better over time without treatment. Despite these limitations, the results were encouraging enough to proceed with a controlled clinical trial of IPT-A.

Controlled Clinical Trial

Data collection for the controlled clinical trial was recently completed. The experimental and control treatment groups each contained 24 patients.

Therapist training consisted of two components: a didactic seminar using the training manual (Mufson et al. 1993) and a clinical practicum. This training was designed to modify the practices of fully trained child and adolescent clinicians to conform to IPT-A, not to train participants to become therapists. Following completion of the didactic program, the therapists entered the clinical practicum. Each participant consecutively treated two cases for 12 weeks each. All sessions were videotaped and discussed in supervision that occurred weekly for 1 hour. Therapists' videotapes were also reviewed by clinical IPT experts who decided whether the participants were competent to be certified as IPT-A therapists. Rating forms designed for the NIMH collaborative study were used to document the competency criteria.

The experimental treatment group was treated with IPT-A,

and the control group was a nonscheduled treatment group. The latter, which has been used in controlled clinical trials for the treatment of acute depression in adults, is discussed in the literature as an ethical control group (DiMascio et al. 1979; Richman et al. 1980). The patients were evaluated using the same measures as in the open clinical trial at weeks 0, 2, 4, 6, 8, 10, and 12. Therapists videotaped their sessions, and the videotapes were regularly reviewed to ensure against therapist drift from the prescribed treatment. The goal of the project was to gain experience and efficacy data on treating depressed adolescents with IPT.

Preliminary Results

Preliminary data suggest that IPT-A may be an effective treatment for depressed adolescents. Despite a relatively small sample, data showed a greater decrease in depressive symptomatology and more signs of improved social functioning and specific problem-solving skills in the IPT-A than in control group patients. There was significantly less attrition in the IPT-A group, suggesting that patients found it an acceptable treatment. The data appear to warrant further investigation on the efficacy of IPT-A compared with other treatment modalities and other adolescent populations.

Summary and Recommendations

The goal in adapting IPT for depressed adolescents and conducting efficacy studies is to add to the small body of research available on psychosocial treatments for depressed adolescents and to develop an effective intervention to treat a serious mental illness in adolescents. The psychopharmacological literature is equivocal, which makes psychosocial treatment development all the more important. However, one needs to keep in mind that even when efficacious medications are available for the treatment of depression in adolescents, there will always be patients for whom medication may not be an option for other medical reasons or those who simply prefer psychosocial treatment over medication. Therefore, it is necessary to develop a variety of efficacious treatment modalities where possible, so that there are always nonmedication alternatives. Based on our experiences, in both an open clinical trial and controlled clinical trial, more studies using IPT-A are warranted to replicate the current findings and to better inform clinicians about treatment efficacy and patient characteristics. IPT-A does not create new therapeutic techniques but rather seeks to organize them in an effective, brief treatment package. As such, while more efficacy data is awaited, it is likely that therapists may find many of the strategies beneficial to the treatment of depressed adolescents in their clinical practice.

References

American Psychiatric Association: Diagnostic and Statistical Manual of Mental Disorders, 3rd Edition, Revised. Washington, DC, American Psychiatric Association, 1987

Brent DA, Holder D, Kolko D, et al: A clinical psychotherapy trial for adolescent depression comparing cognitive, family and supportive therapy. Arch Gen Psychiatry 54:877–885, 1997

Browne A, Finkelhor D: Impact of child sexual abuse: a review of research. Psychopharmacol Bull 99:66–77, 1986

Carroll BJ, Fielding JM, Blashki TG: Depression rating scales: a critical review. Arch Gen Psychiatry 28:361–366, 1973

Chaput F, Moreau D, Mufson L: Depression, in Comprehensive Adolescent Health Care, 2nd Edition. Edited by Friedman SB, Fisher MF, Schouburg SK, et al. St. Louis, MO, Mosby, 1997

DiMascio A, Klerman GL, Weissman MM, et al: A control group for psychotherapy research in acute depression: one solution to ethical and methodological issues. J Psychiatr Res 15:189–197, 1979

Elkin I, Shea MT, Watkins JT, et al: National Institute of Mental Health Treatment of Depression Collaborative Research Program: general effectiveness of treatments. Arch Gen Psychiatry 46:971–982, 1989

Emslie GJ, Rush AJ, Weinberg WA, et al: A double-blind randomized placebo-controlled trial of fluoxetine in depressed children and adolescents. Arch Gen Psychiatry (in press)

Erikson EH: Identity, Youth, and Crisis. New York, WW Norton, 1968

Frank E, Kupfer DF, Perel JM, et al: Three-year outcomes for maintenance therapies in recurrent depression. Arch Gen Psychiatry 47:1093–1099, 1990

Garber J, Kriss MR, Koch M, et al: Recurrent depression in adolescents: a follow-up study. J Am Acad Child Adolesc Psychiatry 27:49–54, 1988

Harrington R, Fudge H, Rutter M, et al: Adult outcomes of childhood and adolescent depression. Arch Gen Psychiatry 46:465–473, 1990

Hersen M, Van Hasselt VB: Behavior Therapy With Children and Adolescents: A Clinical Approach. New York, Wiley, 1987

Jacobson G, Jacobson DS: Impact of marital dissolution on adults and children: the significance of loss and continuity, in The Psychology of Separation and Loss: Perspectives on Development, Life Transitions, and Clinical Practice. Edited by Bloom-Feshbach J, Bloom-Feshbach S. San Francisco, CA, Jossey-Bass, 1987, pp 316–344

Kandel DB, Davies M: Adult sequelae of adolescent depressive symptoms. Arch Gen Psychiatry 43:255–262, 1986

Keller MB, Beardslee WR, Lavori PW, et al: Course of major depression in nonreferred adolescents: a retrospective study. J Affective Disord 15:235–243, 1988

Keller MB, Lavori PW, Beardslee WR, et al: Depression in children and adolescents: new data on "undertreatment" and a literature review on the efficacy of available treatments. J Affective Disord 21:163–171, 1991

Klerman GL, DiMascio A, Weissman MM, et al: Treatment of depression by drugs and psychotherapy. Am J Psychiatry 131:186–194, 1974

Klerman GL, Weissman MM, Rounsaville BH, et al: Interpersonal Psychotherapy of Depression. New York, Basic Books, 1984

Kovacs M, Feinberg TL, Crouse-Novak MA, et al: Depressive disorders in childhood, I: a longitudinal prospective study of characteristics and recovery. Arch Gen Psychiatry 41:229–237, 1984

Kramer AD, Feiguine RJ: Clinical effects of amitriptyline in adolescent depression: a pilot study. J Am Acad Child Adolesc Psychiatry 20:636–644, 1981

Krupnick J: Bereavement during childhood and adolescence, in Bereavement: Reactions, Consequences, and Care. Edited by Osterweis M, Solomon F, Green M. Washington, DC, National Academy Press, 1984, pp 99–141

Kye C, Ryan N: Pharmacologic treatment of child and adolescent depression. Child and Adolescent Psychiatric Clinics of North America 4:261–281, 1995

Lewinsohn PM, Clarke GN, Hops H, et al: Cognitive-behavioral treatment for depressed adolescents. Behavior Therapy 21:385–401, 1990

McCarthy JB: Resistance and countertransference in child and adolescence psychotherapy. Am J Psychoanal 49, 1989

Meyer A: Psychobiology: A Science of Man. Springfield, IL, Charles C Thomas, 1957

Miller D: Adolescence: Psychology, Psychopathology, Psychotherapy. New York, Jason Aronson, 1974

Mufson L, Fairbanks J: Interpersonal psychotherapy for depressed adolescents: a one-year naturalistic follow-up study. J Am Acad Child Adolesc Psychiatry 35:1145–1155, 1996

Mufson L, Moreau D, Weissman MM, et al: Interpersonal Psychotherapy for Depressed Adolescents. New York, Guilford, 1993

Mufson L, Moreau D, Weissman MM, et al: The modification of interpersonal psychotherapy with depressed adolescents (IPT-A): phase I and phase II studies. J Am Acad Child Adolesc Psychiatry 33:695–705, 1994

Raphael B: The Anatomy of Bereavement. New York, Basic Books, 1983

Reich J, Neenan P: Principles common to different short-term psychotherapies. Am J Psychother 40:62–69, 1986

Reynolds WM, Coats KI: A comparison of cognitive-behavioral and relaxation training for the treatment of depression in adolescents. J Consult Clin Psychol 44:653–660, 1980

Reynolds WM, Imber S: Maintenance Therapies in Late-Life Depression (MH#43832). Washington, DC, National Institute of Mental Health, 1988

Richman J, Weissman MM, Klerman GL, et al: Ethical Issues in Clinical Trials: Psychotherapy Research in Acute Depression, Vol 2. New York, Hastings Center, Institute of Society, Ethics, and the Life Sciences, 1980

Robbins DR, Alessi NE, Colfer MV: Treatment of adolescents with major depression: implications of the DST and the melancholic clinical subtype. J Affective Disord 17:99–104, 1989

Rutter M, Tizard J, Yule W, et al: Isle of Wight studies 1964–1974. Psychol Med 6:313–332, 1976

Ryan ND, Puig-Antich J, Cooper T, et al: Imipramine in adolescent major depression: plasma level and clinical response. Acta Psychiatr Scand 73:275–288, 1986

Seigel WM, Golden NH, Gough JW, et al: Depression, self-esteem, and life events in adolescents with chronic disease. J Adolesc Health 11:501–504, 1990

Shaffer D, Garland A, Gould M, et al: Preventing teenage suicide: a critical review. J Am Acad Child Adolesc Psychiatry 27:675–687, 1988

Sifneos PE: Short term dynamic psychotherapy: its history, its impact, and its future. Psychother Psychosom 35:224–229, 1981

Sloane RB, Stapes FR, Schneider LS: Interpersonal therapy versus nortriptyline for depression in the elderly, in Clinical and Pharmacological Studies in Psychiatric Disorders. Edited by Burrows GD, Norman TR, Dennerstein L. London, John Libbey, 1985, pp 344–346

Strober M: Depressive illness in adolescence. Psychiatric Annals 15:375–378, 1985

Strober M, Lampert C, Schmidt S, et al: The course of major depressive disorder in adolescents, I: recovery and risk of manic switching in a follow-up of psychotic and nonpsychotic subtypes. J Am Acad Child Adolesc Psychiatry 32:34–42, 1993

Sullivan HS: Clinical Studies in Psychiatry. New York, WW Norton, 1956

Swift WJ, Wonderlich SA: Interpretation of transference in the psychotherapy of adolescents and young adults. J Am Acad Child Adolesc Psychiatry 29:929–936, 1990

Weissman MM: Mastering Depression: A Patient's Guide to Interpersonal Psychotherapy. Albany, NY, Graywind, 1995, pp 1–78

Weissman MM, Klerman GL, Paykel ES, et al: Treatment effects on the social adjustment of depressed patients. Arch Gen Psychiatry 30:771–778, 1974

Weissman MM, Prusoff BA, DiMascio A, et al: The efficacy of drugs and psychotherapy in the treatment of acute depressive episodes. Am J Psychiatry 136:555–558, 1979

Weissman MM, Rounsaville BJ, Chevron ES: Training psychotherapists to participate in psychotherapy outcome studies: identifying and dealing with the research requirement. Am J Psychiatry 139:1442–1446, 1982

Welner A, Welner Z, Fishman R: Psychiatric adolescent inpatients: eight- to ten-year follow-up. Arch Gen Psychiatry 36:698–700, 1979

Whitaker A, Johnson J, Shaffer D, et al: Uncommon troubles in young people: prevalence estimates of selected psychiatric disorders in a nonreferred adolescent population. Arch Gen Psychiatry 47:487–496, 1990

Wilkes TCR, Belsher G, Rush AJ, et al: Cognitive Therapy for Depressed Adolescents. New York, Guilford, 1994

Chapter 3

Maintenance Interpersonal Psychotherapy: A Preventive Treatment for Depression

Cynthia Spanier, Ph.D., and Ellen Frank, Ph.D.

Several forms of preventive treatment have shown promise in improving the long-term course of recurrent unipolar depression. In this chapter we focus exclusively on maintenance interpersonal psychotherapy (IPT-M) (Frank 1991), a nonpharmacological *interpersonal* approach to preventing the recurrence of major depression. Interpersonal psychotherapy (IPT) focuses on the association between the onset and persistence of depression and *current* acute or long-term interpersonal stressors. As a present-oriented interpersonal approach to the treatment and prevention of depression, IPT considers the social environment a particularly important domain in the onset, maintenance, and course of depression.

IPT was originally developed in a research context as part of a clinical maintenance treatment trial beginning in 1968 (Klerman et al. 1974; Weissman et al. 1974). This study examined the effects of 8 months of psychotherapy in comparison with continued pharmacotherapy in depressed women who had remitted

This research was supported in part by grants from the National Institute of Mental Health to Ellen Frank (Maintenance Therapies in Recurrent Depression, MH29618, and Maintenance Psychotherapy in Recurrent Depression, MH49115), David Kupfer (Mental Health Clinical Research Center for the Study of Affective Disorders, MH30915), and Paul Pilkonis (Clinical Research Training for Psychologists, MH18269).

following 6–8 weeks of amitriptyline therapy. This was the first efficacy study of IPT, and by today's standards, it fit the model of a continuation study. It was also the only controlled trial reported in the literature examining the *protective* capacity of psychotherapy (Frank 1991).

Since this initial clinical trial, IPT has emerged as a standardized, empirically validated treatment for the acute and preventive treatment of major depressive disorder (see Frank and Spanier [1995], Frank et al. [1993], Prochaska and Norcross [1994], and Weissman and Markowitz [1994] for reviews). As one of the promising forms of psychosocial treatment for depression, IPT has shown consistent efficacy in a series of well-designed acute (DiMascio et al. 1979; Elkin et al. 1989), continuation (Klerman et al. 1974), and maintenance (Frank et al. 1990) treatment trials. Thus, in addition to being an efficacious short-term treatment, maintenance IPT, or IPT-M (Frank 1991), has been particularly useful in reducing the risk of recurrence in patients with recurrent unipolar depression.

That IPT was originally developed for preventing relapse following recovery from a pharmacologically treated acute episode is interesting since the importance of prevention in mood disorders has received widespread acceptance only in the last decade. This early relapse prevention treatment trial, begun more than 25 years ago, reflected Klerman's understanding 1) that major depression follows a chronic or recurrent course for most individuals, 2) that the critical problem in the treatment of depression is the prevention of relapse and recurrence, and 3) of the need to develop and test both pharmacological and nonpharmacological treatments that reduce the risk of recurrence.

Fifteen years following the start of the original clinical trial of IPT, IPT-M was developed as a psychotherapeutic treatment to specifically address the critical problem of recurrence in patients who had fully recovered from an acute episode of depression. Like the original prophylactic trial of IPT, we developed IPT-M in a research context, as part of the Pittsburgh study of Maintenance Therapies in Recurrent Depression (MTRD) carried out between 1982 and 1989 (Frank et al. 1990). This protocol was the first 3-year study examining the protective capacity of IPT-M, alone and in combination with medication.

We begin this chapter by discussing the innovations involved in developing maintenance IPT as a treatment for the prevention of depression. These innovations are based on the work of Klerman and colleagues, who developed IPT specifically for the acute treatment of outpatients with depression. After describing IPT in its maintenance treatment form relative to IPT in its acute treatment form, we review the empirical evidence that validates its efficacy as a preventive treatment of recurrent depression. IPT has been tested in two prophylactic studies; both indicated that IPT is superior to a no-treatment condition, medication clinic, and placebo. In considering who is maximally protected by IPT-M, we review biological, psychological, and clinical correlates associated with enhanced response to IPT-M. Finally, we highlight future directions for IPT-M and propose hypothesized protective mechanisms of maintenance IPT.

IPT-M for Prevention of Depression

Overview and Description of IPT-M

Similar to IPT, the development and pilot testing of IPT-M involved a rigorous methodology designed to meet requirements for testing a psychotherapy in a controlled clinical trial. The first step was to write a pilot treatment manual outlining the differences between IPT and the planned IPT-M. In this treatment manual, the adaptation of IPT to a maintenance treatment for the prevention of depression was based extensively on IPT as developed by Klerman and colleagues (1984) (Frank 1991). In addition to writing a treatment manual, treatments were standardized and monitored during the pilot testing period. Therapists met weekly in group supervision to discuss videotaped pilot IPT-M sessions with Cleon Cornes, M.D., who had been certified as an IPT trainer by the originators of IPT, the Yale University supervisors. Each therapist had been certified as an IPT therapist based on a criterion evaluation of his or her videotaped pilot session by the IPT trainer. In addition, all sessions were audiotaped and then rated by objective raters for treatment adherence to the techniques and strategies of IPT. All therapists were thoroughly familiarized with the therapeutic goals of IPT-M.

Similarities Between IPT and IPT-M

Many similarities exist between IPT and IPT-M. Both IPT and IPT-M are manual-based treatments focusing on the analysis of social roles and on the resolution of current interpersonal problems. Similar to IPT, during the actual practice of IPT-M, the therapist focuses on helping the patient to master current social roles and improve interpersonal relations. Analysis and reconstruction of intrapsychic or cognitive events from the past are not the focus, although both IPT and IPT-M therapists acknowledge the profound impact of early developmental experiences and unconscious intrapsychic wishes and conflicts on later patterns of interpersonal relationships. Instead, it is assumed that early childhood experiences will be reflected in the patient's *current* social roles and patterns of relating in relationships. Thus, the focus is on current social dilemmas.

IPT-M (Frank 1991) also preserves the four problem areas of IPT: role transitions, interpersonal role disputes, interpersonal deficits, and grief. In addition, it implements the strategies that distinguish IPT (e.g., linking the onset of symptoms to disputes with significant others in the patient's current social arena and exploration and clarification of feelings associated with loss of a role) and the techniques of IPT (e.g., elicitation of feelings, nonjudgmental exploration of the affective quality of relationships, and behavior change techniques to foster the development of satisfying and adaptive interpersonal behaviors).

Differences Between IPT and IPT-M

IPT-M differs from IPT in its goals, number of problem areas addressed, and timing. The primary goal of IPT-M is to prevent recurrence (i.e., sustain wellness) in patients who are fully remitted; in contrast, the goal of IPT is to bring about remission in patients who are in the midst of an acute episode of depression. Moreover, IPT-M is designed to treat patients in a maintenance format for several years (patients were treated for up to 3 years with IPT-M in the MTRD study (Frank et al. 1990). Accordingly, the number of problem areas typically focused on with a patient in IPT-M is greater than in IPT for the acute treatment of depression. Given the long course of IPT-M, IPT-M therapists have the opportunity to focus on "long-standing patterns of interpersonal behavior which appear to be non-adaptive for the patient" (Frank 1991, p. 262). However, they do not attempt personality reconstruction, as is done in traditional psychoanalysis.

Since the goal of IPT-M is prevention, the therapist is mindful of the early development of interpersonal problems similar to those associated with the onset of the patient's most recent episode, as well as earlier episodes, of depression. The emphasis in IPT-M is on augmenting the patient's strengths and helping him or her assume much of the responsibility for the prevention of future episodes. Thus, the patient is also encouraged to be watchful for the appearance of early somatic and cognitive symptoms characteristic of prior depressive episodes. If symptoms are reported, strategies are planned and implemented by the therapist and patient to prevent the onset of a new episode. Consistent with an interpersonal approach to the treatment of depression, these strategies are primarily interpersonal in emphasis and intended to improve the patient's mood and functioning (e.g., increasing integration in supportive social networks so that others are available for support and to aid in coping with stressful life events, identifying and attending to one's own needs, and focusing less on the needs of others).

Although the techniques and strategies used in IPT-M are similar to those in IPT, the time frame of IPT-M places a relatively greater emphasis on developing strategies to prevent future interpersonal difficulties (e.g., developing adaptive coping strategies in preparation for an upcoming and potentially stressful interpersonal event). However, like IPT, a predominant here-

and-now, present-oriented focus is maintained in IPT-M (Spanier 1997). At the same time, it is important to point out that IPT and IPT-M are not conducted in an interpersonal time vacuum. Even though analysis of events from the past is not a focus during the actual practice of IPT-M, an interpersonal inventory is taken at the start of IPT. During the inventory, the IPT therapist systematically reviews the history of the patient's current and past important relationships and social roles within those relationships "to get a full picture of what the important current social interactions are in the patient's life" (Klerman et al. 1984, p. 86). In sum, although a focus on the present and future appears to be important in IPT-M, this focus has a context that is anchored in the patient's interpersonal history.

IPT-M, in contrast to weekly IPT for acute treatment, was scheduled once per month (Frank et al. 1990). This modification in the timing of IPT sessions was justified in accordance with the nature of the study population, which consisted of asymptomatic patients with a history of recurrent episodes of depression. In addition, provision of monthly therapy sessions appeared congruous with the primary goal of IPT-M (i.e., prevention of a new episode of depression). Although monthly IPT sessions showed a significant effect in extending the interval between depressive episodes (as will be discussed shortly), it may be that more frequent contact, weekly or biweekly, could have produced an even better outcome, especially in patients who preferred more frequent contact or who experienced loss or increased anxiety by moving from weekly IPT to monthly IPT-M. A clinical trial is currently under way to test the efficacy of weekly, biweekly, and monthly IPT-M. The goal of this investigation is to maximize the preventive capacity of IPT-M by establishing the ideal contact frequency. Clearly, at least for a subset of patients in the MTRD protocol, moving from weekly to monthly contact was the optimal preventive strategy: "These individuals seemed able to benefit from the longer distance between therapy sessions as a direct consequence of having had more time between sessions to think about and observe the interpersonal context of their lives and to experiment with new interpersonal behaviors" (Frank 1991, p. 264).

In IPT, typically one problem area (or occasionally two areas) becomes the focus of therapy during the 16 weeks of acute treatment. In contrast, in IPT-M, two to three problem areas typically are addressed given its application as a 3-year course of treatment. The problem areas that become the focus of treatment usually involve a combination of role transitions, role disputes, interpersonal deficits, and less frequently grief issues, unless a significant loss-related event occurs during maintenance treatment (Frank et al. 1993). Identification of the problem area in IPT-M evolves over the course of acute treatment, during which a number of interpersonal themes surface but are not the focus. These themes, particularly ingrained interpersonal patterns that continue to be problematic for the patient during remission or as a result of remission, are noted by the therapist and explored in IPT-M: "The long course of IPT-M provides a secure base from which patients can experiment with new interpersonal styles and to which they can bring their questions and concerns about the success of the experimentation into the therapy" (Frank 1991, p. 263).

Summary of IPT-M for Prevention of Depression

IPT-M was designed specifically to maintain recovery and reduce vulnerability to future episodes of depression by improving social adjustment. Thus, the focus in IPT-M is on the interpersonal and psychosocial context of the well state, and a central goal of this focus is to prevent or mitigate interpersonal stress. Accordingly, it was hypothesized that the risk of recurrence would be reduced in IPT-M by improving social adjustment; the patient would be helped to cope more effectively with interpersonal and social problems associated with the well state, which would in turn reduce the number and severity of stressful life events. This decreased stress consequently would reduce the risk of recurrence. In the next section, we briefly outline the theoretical and empirical bases of IPT that have provided support for the hypothesized protective mechanisms of IPT-M as stated earlier. In this case, the theoretical bases for IPT and IPT-M are supported by a substantial body of empirical evidence linking interpersonal adversities to depression.

Theoretical and Empirical Bases for an Interpersonal Approach in the Treatment and Prevention of Depression

IPT and thus IPT-M are based on an interpersonal approach to psychotherapy, founded in the United States with Adolf Meyer's psychobiological approach to psychiatric illness. Meyer, who was strongly influenced by Darwin, accentuated the patient's current interpersonal relations and social experiences and conceptualized psychopathology to be the expression of a patient's attempt to adapt to the ever-changing psychosocial environment. Meyer's approach emphasized that both "normal" and "abnormal" behaviors represent adaptations to the social environment and ways of coping with distressing interpersonal situations.

Harry Stack Sullivan, who studied under Meyer, continued this work and is known for articulating the theory of interpersonal relations and emphasizing an interpersonal approach to the understanding of depression. Sullivan (1953) assumed a link between interpersonal processes and the etiopathogenesis of mental illness. He believed that much of human behavior was influenced by the need for reciprocal and mutually satisfying personal relationships and thus argued that the area of psychotherapeutic focus be on the patient's current interpersonal relations. Accordingly, disturbances in interpersonal relations, in this view, are both antecedents to and consequences of mental illness (Klerman et al. 1984).

In addition to these theories, a major theoretical source for understanding depression in an interpersonal context comes from J. Bowlby's theory of attachment. Bowlby proposed that the infant and the mothering figure, as well as human beings in general, have an instinctive propensity to form strong affectional bonds to preferred others and that an unwilling separation from or loss of these attachment bonds leads to various forms of emotional distress including anxiety, anger, despair, depression, and emotional detachment (Bowlby 1982). Bowlby (1977a, 1977b) also suggested that many forms of psychopathology are the results of an inability to form or maintain emotional bonds. Attachment theory has provided a solid basis for understanding an interpersonal approach to depression and for developing psychotherapeutic strategies designed to change maladaptive interpersonal patterns generated by unsatisfactory attachments in childhood.

IPT and IPT-M emphasize the psychosocial and interpersonal context associated with the onset, persistence, and course of mood episodes. Even a brief review of the empirical evidence linking interpersonal difficulties in the current social environment with clinical depression strongly supports this association. Aspects of the social environment have been shown to increase vulnerability to the negative impact of stressful life events and thus also to the onset or recurrence of depression. The structural aspects of social networks (inadequate social attachments or general supports), functional aspects of social supports (lack of confiding, emotionally supportive relationships and lack of intimacy), and antecedent life events and long-term interpersonal stressors, especially those involving loss and disappointment, have all been shown to be associated with the onset of depression. Thus, close personal relations and satisfactory social supports are important aspects of the social environment that protect against depression, and disruption of these attachments plays a significant role in the development of depression, especially when exposed to stressful life events (see Frank and Spanier 1995 for a review).

In addition, depression itself is a stressful life event that influences interpersonal relationships. Thus, the interpersonal consequences of depression—persistent deficits in social adjustment—increase a patient's vulnerability to a recurrence of depression by their likelihood of leading to loss-related life events and ongoing distress (e.g., disruption of close relationships, separation, divorce, and withdrawal from social networks and activities).

Summary of Theoretical and Empirical Bases of IPT in the Prevention of Depression

In sum, IPT-M is a system of psychotherapy incorporating the theoretical positions of Meyer, Sullivan, and Bowlby, as well as the empirical evidence linking difficulties in the immediate social environment with the onset and pathogenesis of depression. Based on the empirical evidence and our own clinical experience in applying IPT-M in recurrent depression, we feel justified in concluding that maintenance of recovery and reduced vulnerability to a recurrence of depression in IPT-M is related to a focus on improving the quality of a patient's current social network and mastery of social roles. These goals are achieved particularly by helping the patient to develop more productive strategies for coping with interpersonal distress.

Does IPT Prevent Recurrence? Review of Results

Two randomized, controlled trials have been completed that demonstrate the efficacy of IPT as a preventive treatment for major depression. In the original relapse prevention study of IPT (i.e., the New Haven–Boston Collaborative Study of the Treatment of Acute Depression), Klerman et al. (1974) assessed the effect of IPT in an 8-month, six-cell trial in 150 depressed female outpatients who had responded with symptom reduction to 4–6 weeks of amitriptyline therapy. Patients were randomly assigned to 8 months of weekly IPT, medication, IPT and medication, IPT and placebo, placebo alone, or no treatment. At the conclusion of treatment, relapse rates were highest for patients receiving no treatment (36%) as compared with the other three active treatment groups (medication alone [12%], IPT alone [16.7%], and the combined IPT and medication group [12.5%]). Patients receiving IPT demonstrated improved social functioning, although these effects were not apparent for 6–8 months (Weissman et al. 1974).

The investigators concluded that superior outcomes were produced by the combination of IPT with medication. However, the design of the study, in which medication initially was administered alone, restricts generalizations regarding the efficacy of IPT to patients who have already responded positively to imipramine. The small sample size in each cell (approximately $n = 25$ subjects), which reduced the power to detect statistically significant differences despite that fact that several appear to have clinical significance, further limits conclusions regarding the efficacy of IPT. Moreover, the delivery of psychotherapy was, at that time, relatively unstandardized, and the data analytic approach did not use survival methods considered most appropriate for the analysis of follow-up data (Greenhouse et al. 1989; Singer and Willett 1991).

The second study, the 3-year Pittsburgh MTRD study (Frank et al. 1990; Kupfer et al. 1992), is the longest randomized maintenance trial to date. In depressed patients who showed a clear history of repeated episodes of depression, Frank et al. (1990) contrasted IPT-M with maintenance pharmacotherapy (imipramine), combination pharmacotherapy and psychotherapy, and a control group in a five-cell design to determine whether IPT-M alone or in combination with medication could play a significant role in the prevention of recurrence.

In this trial all subjects were treated acutely with a combination of IPT and imipramine (imipramine hydrochloride, 150–300 mg, four times per day). Initial treatment was provided weekly for 12 weeks, every other week for the next 8 weeks, and then monthly until patients' symptoms diminished to a remission range defined as a Hamilton Rating Scale for Depression (HRSD) (Hamilton 1960) score <7 and a Raskin (Raskin et al. 1969) score <5. Once stabilized, patients continued to received both IPT and imipramine until they had demonstrated evidence of sustained remission (i.e., HRSD <7 or Raskin <5 for 20 weeks), a unique feature of this study.

Following this period of short-term and continuation treatment, the experimental maintenance phase began. The 128 patients who achieved a sustained remission of their acute depressive episode were randomly assigned to one of the five maintenance treatments: 1) IPT-M alone, 2) IPT-M with placebo tablet, 3) IPT-M with imipramine, 4) medication clinic visits with imipramine, or 5) medication clinic visits with placebo tablet. Maintenance treatment sessions occurred monthly for 3 years or until the patient experienced a recurrence of illness. In addition, patients underwent sleep electroencephalographic (EEG) monitoring at baseline and periodically throughout the course of treatment, and thus biological variables such as delta sleep ratio, rapid eye movement (REM) latency, and slow-wave sleep percentage were incorporated as part of this treatment research.

In contrast with previous studies, imipramine was maintained at the highest dose of medication ever employed in a maintenance trial (mean dose >200 mg/day) rather than being tapered from acute treatment levels, and IPT was administered monthly and thus at the lowest dose ever in comparison with other clinical trials. Results of survival analyses showed that active imipramine, maintained at an average dose of 208 mg/day, provided a prophylactic effect to a larger proportion of patients over a longer period of time than in any previous study of maintenance therapy of recurrent depression (Frank et al. 1990). Of most relevance here, we also demonstrated that when patients received a combination of pharmacotherapy and IPT for the treatment of their acute episode, those who continued to receive IPT on a monthly basis following drug discontinuation remained well significantly longer than those who did not. The mean survival time was 45 weeks for the medication clinic and placebo group, 74 weeks for the IPT-M and placebo group, 82 weeks for the IPT-M alone group, 124 weeks for the medication clinic and imipramine group, and 131 weeks for the IPT-M and active imipramine group.

These results show a clinically meaningful and statistically significant effect for maintenance IPT, even when limited to monthly contact, among patients with highly recurrent forms of major depression. In conclusion, this long-term outcome study clearly established the value of maintenance IPT in the prevention of recurrence in major depression.

Taken together, the results from the MTRD study and the original relapse prevention study by Klerman et al. (1974) provide an impressive record of success and attest to the efficacy of IPT in the prevention of clinical depression. The performance of

IPT in these clinical trials consistently surpasses no treatment and placebo therapy in the maintenance treatment of outpatients with depression.

Variables Moderating the Efficacy of Maintenance IPT Following Discontinuation of Pharmacotherapy: Clinical and Psychobiological Correlates of Outcome

In addition to examining the efficacy of preventive treatments, another overarching aim of this clinical trial was to identify and better understand potential risk and protective factors influencing the efficacy (i.e., response or nonresponse) to preventive treatments. Although much research has examined treatment response to pharmacotherapy, the purpose of this work was to identify and integrate psychological and biological processes that work to optimize response to psychotherapy. By examining more closely which variables moderate the effect of long-term preventive treatment of depression (in this case, IPT) after patients discontinue pharmacotherapy, we hoped to 1) advance our knowledge regarding ways to maximize the preventive capacity of IPT and 2) increase our understanding of ways to match patients to treatment, be they psychotherapeutic, pharmacological, or both. Consistent with the integrative approach used in this long-term treatment trial, both biological and psychosocial correlates have been examined.

Biological Correlates of Long-Term Outcome: EEG Sleep Parameters

EEG sleep changes are a consistent biological finding in patients with recurrent major depression. In earlier studies we had identified EEG sleep correlates of acute response to pharmacotherapy and psychotherapy. In addition, numerous studies have characterized a depressive episode with respect to specific EEG findings (see Buysse and Kupfer 1993 for a review). In this project of

---

long-term preventive treatment, we also identified EEG sleep parameters that were associated with sustained recovery. We found that delta sleep ratio, which represents the proportional distribution of delta (i.e., slow-wave) EEG sleep in the first and second non-REM (NREM) sleep periods, was highly predictive of the length of survival following discontinuation of drug treatment (Kupfer et al. 1990). Specifically, Kupfer et al. (1990) found that decreased slow-wave or delta sleep early in the night was associated with earlier recurrence during maintenance treatment. In contrast with depressed individuals, who tend to show reduced delta sleep in the first rather than second NREM sleep period, nondepressed individuals show a linear decrease in delta sleep throughout the night (Frank et al. 1993).

Since we had noted a significant influence of monthly psychotherapy on length of survival, we also examined response to maintenance psychotherapy in relation to delta sleep ratio, seeking to integrate biological measures with psychotherapeutic treatment. We found that patients who received IPT-M and had normal delta sleep in the first NREM period (i.e., high delta ratio) survived significantly longer. In contrast, patients with decreased delta sleep in the first NREM period were not significantly protected by monthly IPT-M. Thus, normal delta sleep was identified as a biological correlate associated with enhanced response to psychotherapy, in this case IPT-M, whereas decreased delta sleep was associated with a higher risk of recurrence.

Psychological Correlates of Outcome

Treatment Specificity

We also ascertained whether higher-quality IPT was associated with longer survival (Frank et al. 1991). In an effort to further understand the relationship between monthly psychotherapy and longer survival time, Frank et al. (1991) examined the contribution of treatment quality and demographic and clinical variables to long-term survival with IPT-M alone and IPT-M plus placebo conditions. Treatment quality was defined as the extent to which therapists conformed to specific principles, goals, and techniques of IPT, thus labeled treatment specificity. It tested even more rigorously the efficacy of IPT-M and thus provided further evidence to support the earlier conclusion of a specific prophylactic effect for IPT-M.

Although no demographic or clinical variables were related to long-term survival in the maintenance IPT conditions in this follow-up report, higher (i.e., above the median) specificity of IPT-M was associated with significantly increased survival time, with a median survival time of almost 2 years (102 weeks, SE = 8 weeks, $P < .001$; see Figure 3–1). In contrast, patient-therapist dyads rated as having low treatment specificity of IPT-M, or who, in other words, were unable to focus consistently on interpersonal concerns, had a median survival time of less than

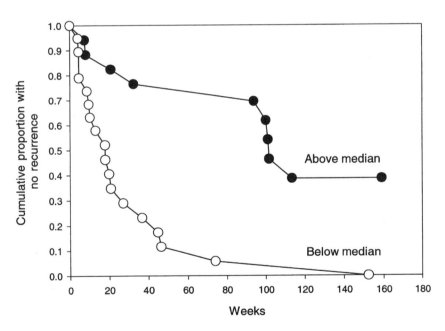

Figure 3–1. Weeks of recurrence based on Therapy Rating Scale—interpersonal score.
Source. Reprinted from Frank E, Kupfer DJ, Wagner EF, et al.: "Efficacy of Interpersonal Psychotherapy as a Maintenance Treatment of Recurrent Depression: Contributing Factors." *Arch Gen Psychiatry* 48:1053–1059, 1991. Copyright 1991 American Medical Association. Used with permission.

5 months (18 weeks, SE = 4.6 weeks). Patients in the low-specificity dyads received no more protection from the IPT-M treatment assignment than was provided by the medication clinic plus placebo assignment (median survival time was 21 weeks). We concluded that when patients are able to maintain a consistent focus on interpersonal issues, monthly sessions of IPT provide substantial protection against recurrence of depression.

Interestingly, these results are consistent with data drawn from the original relapse prevention study of IPT (Klerman et al. 1974) in which "discussion of mental symptoms" and "overt expression of anxiety" were significantly associated with relapse (Jacobson et al. 1977). Also relevant to our understanding of the robust effects of treatment specificity on survival, Jacobson et al. (1977) concluded that the group of patients who relapsed, in focusing primarily on "the self-oriented and static topic of mental symptoms" (p. 145), were thus able to avoid more adaptive work on current interpersonal issues or, in limiting discussion to symptomatic concerns, on what could be done to ameliorate them.

Integrating Biological and Psychological Correlates of Treatment Outcome

What remained unclear given the Kupfer et al. (1990) delta ratio findings and the Frank et al. (1991) treatment specificity findings (which indicated that psychotherapy that was more specifically interpersonal was associated with significantly increased survival time) was how these specific biological and psychological factors, when taken together, were related to treatment outcome as measured by length of survival time without a new episode. Thus, in an effort to integrate biological and psychological correlates of treatment outcome following discontinuation of somatic therapy, we (Spanier et al. 1996) examined the *simultaneous* contribution of delta sleep ratio, a presumably traitlike sleep EEG measure, and treatment specificity of IPT-M in a similar group of patients assigned to IPT-M without active medication.

Analysis of treatment specificity ratings across sessions and delta ratio at baseline indicated that patients survived the longest when both pretreatment delta sleep parameters more closely approximated those of nondepressed individuals and monthly IPT-M was of higher quality (see Figure 3–2). In fact, a 3-year survival rate of 73% for this group did not appear to be significantly different from antidepressant therapy in this study of maintenance treatments for depression. With both vulnerability factors present, none (0%) of the patients survived; in fact, all patients participating in lower-quality IPT-M with reduced delta sleep experienced recurring depression within the first year of the 3-year trial. In contrast, the original outcome survival analysis showed that 35% of the patients randomly assigned to IPT-M survived the full 3 years (Frank et al. 1990). This subsequent analysis shows that in the absence of biological (decreased delta sleep in the first NREM period) or psychotherapeutic (lower-quality therapy) vulnerability factors, survival rates im-

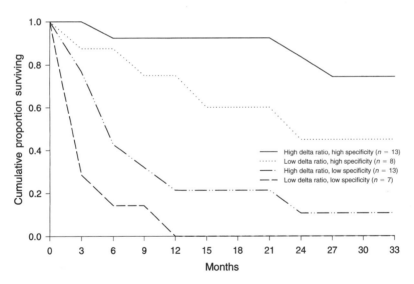

Figure 3–2. Relationship of treatment specificity and delta ratio to time to recurrence.
Source. Spanier CA, Frank E, McEachran AB, et al.: "The Prophylaxis of Depressive Episodes in Recurrent Depression Following Discontinuation of Drug Therapy: Integrating Psychological and Biological Factors." *Psychological Medicine* 26:461–475, 1996. With permission of Cambridge University Press.

prove dramatically (from 0% to 73% survival). When one compares these rates and the original IPT-M outcome survival rates (35% versus 73%), it becomes clear that both the quality of the psychotherapy and the pretreatment sleep parameters, such as normal delta sleep, have highly significant effects for maximizing the preventive capacity of maintenance psychotherapy. For at least a subgroup of patients with recurrent depressive episodes and healthy delta sleep, good-quality monthly IPT-M is a powerful preventive treatment.

Also important was the finding that good-quality IPT-M (i.e., higher specificity of IPT-M) was more effective than poor-quality IPT-M, even in patients with low delta ratios (i.e., markedly abnormal baseline sleep) who were thus biologically vulnerable to recurrence. (Note the 44% 3-year survival rate for patients characterized by decreased delta sleep but whose therapy sessions were rated above average; see Figure 3–2.) This finding suggests that good-quality psychotherapy provides significant protection, even for patients with a biological vulnerability factor for recurrence. Perhaps above-average therapy serves as a buffer, mitigating the negative effects of biological vulnerabilities—in this case, EEG sleep disturbance. At the same time, patients with abnormal sleep profiles were less responsive to good-quality preventive IPT (44% versus 73% survival). What remained unclear was how to identify which patients with reduced delta sleep would be protected by above-average therapy; our findings with respect to patient attitudes helped us to answer this question.

We (Spanier et al. 1996) concluded that at least for a subgroup of patients with recurrent depressive episodes and healthy delta sleep, good-quality monthly IPT is as powerful a preventive treatment as what is now considered the gold standard, antidepressant medication. In addition, these findings modified the earlier finding (Kupfer et al. 1990) of the significant benefit of monthly IPT-M only for patients with high baseline delta ratio but not low delta sleep ratio. The findings from this study showed that high-specificity IPT-M provided significant protection, even for patients with abnormal baseline EEG sleep and thus a biological vulnerability for recurrence. The finding of a 0% survival rate suggests that IPT-M was an ineffective preven-

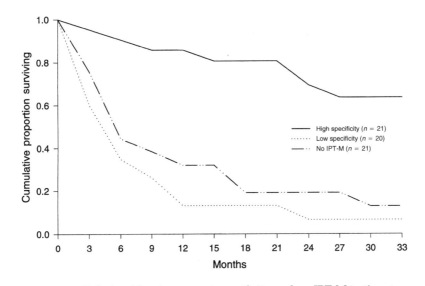

Figure 3–3. Relationship of treatment specificity and no IPT-M to time to recurrence.
Source. Spanier CA, Frank E, McEachran AB, et al.: "The Prophylaxis of Depressive Episodes in Recurrent Depression Following Discontinuation of Drug Therapy: Integrating Psychological and Biological Factors." *Psychological Medicine* 26:461–475, 1996. With permission of Cambridge University Press.

tive treatment for patients characterized by decreased delta sleep who participated in lower-quality therapy. This fact is even more pronounced when one compares survival rates between patients assigned to the medication clinic and pill placebo treatment in the MTRD study (13%) with survival rates in patients participating in low-specificity psychotherapy in the absence of medication (7%) (see Figure 3–3: high-specificity IPT-M group versus the no IPT-M group, $P < .0002$; low-specificity IPT-M group versus no-IPT-M group, $P = .23$).[1] The finding that survival rates between the low-specificity IPT-M and no IPT-M groups are not significantly different suggests that participation in below-

---

[1] We compared subjects ($n = 21$) who were randomly assigned to the medication clinic plus placebo group, and thus did not participate in IPT treatment and were unmedicated, and had delta ratio measurements, with the $n = 41$ IPT-M subjects examined in the Spanier et al. (1996) report.

average therapy is no more effective (in fact, it is less effective clinically) than assignment to the control condition—in this case, no active psychotherapy or medication. These results showed that it is the *quality* of IPT-M rather than simply the *occurrence* of IPT-M that contributes to its preventive capacity.

Therapists

We also examined the association between individual therapists, treatment specificity, and time to recurrence in the group of patients assigned to IPT-M without active medication (Frank et al. 1991; Spanier et al. 1996). We (Spanier et al. 1996) found a significant association between therapist and outcome as measured by time to recurrence in this expanded group of patients receiving IPT-M without medication. Accordingly, the variable clinician was included as a covariate in the primary survival analyses. (Although this finding is in contrast to the previous Frank et al. [1991] report, it was not surprising since a trend effect for therapist [$P = .17$] was previously found and thus was used as a covariate in the original Frank et al. [1991] survival analysis.) However, no differences were found between clinicians on patients' HRSD scores at the index assessment. We concluded that the efficacy of IPT-M was related, in part, to differences in some aspect of therapists' behavior, as yet unknown.[2]

---

[2]The finding that therapists differed in effectiveness in the MTRD study is consistent with previous findings (Crits-Christoph and Mintz 1991; Luborsky et al. 1985; O'Malley et al. 1988; Rounsaville et al. 1987), and, similar to recent investigations, rigorous procedures designed to minimize variability among therapists were implemented at the outset of the study (Frank 1991). Briefly, therapists were first carefully selected and trained to be competent in IPT. Treatments were standardized by implementing a detailed treatment manual for IPT-M. Frank and colleagues established ongoing group supervision and independently monitored treatment adherence using objective ratings. In addition, over the course of the study, it was found that all therapists had excellent records for retaining patients. However, it appears that even these measures cannot eliminate cross-therapist and cross-case variability in the conduct of treatments, since neither therapists nor patients are automatons. Although this study did not identify characteristics of more effective therapists, the earlier studies attempted to relate qualities of therapists to outcome and found that general aspects of the therapist (e.g., therapist exploration, warmth, and friendliness) and specific skillfulness in conducting IPT were significant correlates of outcome (O'Malley et al. 1988; Rounsaville et al. 1987).

Patient Attitudes and Personality

We examined the contribution of several other patient characteristics, including patient attitudes or expectancies and personality, to treatment specificity and time to recurrence to explore further the issue of the patients' contributions to preventive treatment outcome. The question of interest was whether patient attitude and personality parameters would moderate response to maintenance psychotherapy and thus influence the risk of recurrence in the absence of medication in remitted patients.

In several previous MTRD analyses (Bearden et al. 1996; Frank et al. 1987; Pilkonis and Frank 1988), personality functioning was associated with response to acute treatment. Specifically, we have shown that personality functioned as a moderator of response to combined pharmacotherapy and psychotherapy (IPT) among patients in acute episodes of depression. Patients who responded more slowly and inconsistently during their acute-phase treatment evidenced more personality pathology when fully recovered (Frank et al. 1987). In addition, these analyses corroborate extant literature suggesting that the personalities of recovered unipolar patients can be characterized by two prototypes: the dependent, anxiously attached patient and the obsessive-compulsive character (i.e., excessive dependency and excessive autonomy), although the most prevalent among our group of recovered patients were the fearful, anxious personality dimensions. In contrast, personality pathology was not found to be a significant correlate of long-term response to psychotherapy (IPT-M) or pharmacotherapy in the MTRD trial.

We measured patient attitudes using a 20-item Patient Attitudes and Beliefs (PAB) scale developed for the National Institute of Mental Health Treatment of Depression Collaborative Research Program (NIMH TDCRP) (Elkin et al. 1989).[3] This scale was designed to assess patients' beliefs regarding the cause(s) of

---

[3]We measured patient attitudes at three time periods—baseline, continuation, and premaintenance. The results reported here come from the premaintenance evaluations only, when all patients were asymptomatic and had been that way for an extended period (>20 weeks).

their depression along three factors: biological, cognitive, and social.[4] When examining how patient attitudes might influence treatment specificity and risk of recurrence, the three PAB factor scores were not found to have any association with time to recurrence (P = .36 biological, .33 cognitive, and .41 external). However, when the difference between the biological and cognitive plus external scores was examined (Table 3–1), we found a highly significant effect of patient attitudes and expectations on treatment specificity and survival time, although when taken together, treatment specificity was the only variable remaining significantly associated with outcome.[5] Patients with a larger positive difference (i.e., patients who reported that their biological beliefs were greater relative to their cognitive plus external beliefs) demonstrated a shorter time to recurrence. Of particular interest is the finding of a significant association between patient attitudes and treatment specificity.

Consistent with the view that psychotherapy is a process of reciprocal influence between patient and therapist, we (Spanier et al. 1996) concluded that in addition to the influence of therapists, some portion of the therapy process during maintenance treatment is related to the patients' attitudes about their illness. These findings provide empirical evidence for the clinical assumption that both patient and therapist factors are important moderators of response to (preventive) psychotherapy.

The finding of a significant association among therapist, treatment specificity, and outcome, and the absence of any differences among the three clinician types on patients' HSRD scores at the index assessment, suggested that therapists differ in effectiveness and that this degree of effectiveness impacts treatment spec-

---

[4]PAB *biological* items assess the extent to which patients believe that the cause of their illness is related primarily to neurotransmitter dysfunction or genetic factors; for example, "An imbalance of certain substances in my brain is a cause of my problems." *Cognitive* items assess the extent to which patients believe the cause of their depression is due to the way they think about themselves and the world; for example, "Pessimistic attitudes about many things are a cause of my problems." *Social* items assess the extent to which patients believe the cause of their depression is due to factors in their social environment; for example, "Marital or family problems are a cause of my problems."

[5]We computed PAB difference scores for each patient by summing standardized cognitive plus external scores and then subtracting them from biological scores.

Table 3–1. Survival analyses of patient attitudes, treatment specificity, and time to recurrence using the Cox Proportional Model

Patient Attitudes and Beliefs (PAB) scale difference scores and time to recurrence	
PAB difference scores: the difference between biological and cognitive plus external scores	$P < .0006$
PAB difference scores when including the covariates delta ratio and clinician in the model	$P < .0001$
PAB difference scores when including the covariates delta ratio, clinician, and treatment specificity in the model	$P < .14$
Treatment specificity and time to recurrence with PAB difference scores, delta ratio, and clinician in the model	$P < .024$

PAB difference and treatment specificity scores ($r = .31$; $P < .05$; $N = 41$).

ificity of IPT-M and survival time. At the same time, we found an effect of treatment specificity beyond the significant effects of therapists on outcome, suggesting a patient contribution to specificity (i.e., some patients make it easier than others for therapists to achieve or maintain the interpersonal focus). Thus, it is important to note our finding of the significant association among patient attitudes, treatment specificity, and outcome. It may be that patients in the well state who believe (correctly or not) that the cause of their illness is primarily biological, with psychological or social factors (e.g., distorted cognitions or conflictual relationships) of lesser causal importance, make it more difficult for therapists to achieve a consistent focus on interpersonal concerns in IPT-M and that this lowered treatment specificity is in turn reflected in these patients' shorter times to recurrence. In sum, in addition to therapists, patients (in this case, patient attitudes) contribute to treatment specificity, and high treatment specificity or good-quality therapy is reflected in longer times to recurrence.

These findings are consistent with extensive empirical data indicating that patient expectancies and attitudes are significant correlates of successful outcome in psychotherapy (see Stiles et al. 1986 for a review) and may in fact reflect the degree of patient capacity to become actively engaged in the therapeutic interaction. Thus, the role of patient attitudes in the effectiveness of long-term preventive IPT appears to be extremely important by way of their influence on a patient's capacity to become involved in therapy (Spanier et al. 1996). These findings are also consistent with a treatment matching approach to therapy; that is, one option for maximizing the effectiveness of psychotherapy would be to select only patients who evidence a mind-set to actively participate in the therapeutic process. Alternate interventions need to be considered for patients who do not appear willing to engage in long-term preventive psychotherapy or who do not appear able to assume at least some responsibility for change.

Summary of Biological and Psychological Correlates

Taken together, these studies indicate that a variety of patient and therapist characteristics, as well as factors within the patient-therapist dyad (i.e., treatment specificity), contribute to the efficacy of IPT-M. The data from these three reports (Frank et al. 1990, 1991; Spanier et al. 1996) "point to the potential of maintenance psychotherapy for significantly extending the well interval, if not providing complete prophylaxis" (Frank and Kupfer 1994, p. 505).

Future Directions

In the preceding sections, we have reviewed evidence for the protective capacity of IPT-M in delaying or preventing a recurrence of depression. Each of the preventive studies suggests that IPT is superior to a medication clinic and placebo approach in the prevention of new episodes. Although the original relapse prevention trial suggested that weekly IPT was almost as effective as pharmacotherapy or the combination of pharmacotherapy and IPT in the prevention of relapse, the Frank et al. (1990) long-term maintenance trial found monthly IPT-M less effective than pharmacotherapy and IPT in preventing a recurrence of depressive illness. The results of this clinical trial, while promising with respect to the protective capacity of IPT-M, suggested that we focus our efforts on finding ways to maximize the preventive capacity of IPT-M. Subsequently, we identified biological and psychological correlates that were associated with markedly improved response to IPT-M. Both therapist and patient factors, including sleep EEG variables, the quality (i.e., specificity) of IPT-M, patient attitudes, and therapist effectiveness, are related to the efficacy of IPT-M.

The remaining challenges in working with IPT are 1) to understand how IPT exerts its effects, 2) to determine whether there are ways to make IPT even more efficacious than it has already been shown to be, and 3) to test the generalizability of IPT to other populations and other disorders (Frank and Spanier 1995).

How Does IPT Work?

We currently have a number of outcome studies establishing the efficacy of IPT in unipolar depression and several studies exploring critical patient, therapist, and relationship variables affecting the degree of acute and long-term response to IPT. It is important now to refine our understanding of what specific mechanisms in IPT help to reduce symptoms and delay or prevent their return.

We proposed a model of the protective mechanisms of IPT-M in our section summarizing IPT for depression prevention. Thus we propose that IPT-M works by improving the quality of attachment, enhancing social support, and helping the patient to develop more productive strategies for coping with interpersonal and social problems. In turn, improved coping and better social functioning decrease the number and severity of stressful life events, especially those involving loss or disappointment, or at least mitigate or buffer their effects. This model has never been fully tested in IPT-M and warrants further study. One arm of this model, the association between life stress and depression, has consistent empirical support—that is, there is unequivocal agreement in the literature that antecedent life events may play a role in producing, triggering, or maintaining a depression. Our research group, in tandem with Brown, Harris, and colleagues, who have studied the relationship between life stress and depressive episodes for the last 20 years (Bebbington et al. 1988,

1993; Brown and Harris 1978, 1989), found that stressful life events played an important role in the onset of depressive episodes characterized by nonendogenous features (Brown et al. 1994; Frank et al. 1994). Our group is now exploring the relationship among gender, life events, and depression in a currently under way controlled trial testing the prophylactic capacity of IPT-M in women suffering from recurrent depression.

We have also hypothesized other active ingredients of IPT. Even though its theoretical bases lie in the interpersonal and cultural schools, both IPT and IPT-M are practiced as present-oriented therapies, focusing on current here-and-now relationships. It has been assumed that past family of origin work and reconstruction of early developmental experiences are not essential for therapeutic response. A study testing these assumptions with respect to the time orientation of IPT-M has recently been completed, with results to follow (Spanier 1997). One component of the study was based on a hypothesis suggested by the late Dr. Daniel Friedman, who speculated that IPT-M's effect is based on what it does *not* do—that is, encourage rumination about the past. Thus, we hypothesized that among subjects treated with IPT-M, those whose therapy sessions focused most on present and future problems, which by definition precluded obsessive rumination about unalterable negative experiences from the past, were expected to have the best outcome. This hypothesis was also supported by an area of recent research that found that self-focused rumination in people with dysphoria can maintain and exacerbate depressed mood and contribute to pessimistic thinking and poor problem solving ability (Lyubomirsky and Nolen-Hoeksema 1993, 1995).

Our finding of a significant association between individual therapists and outcome suggests that certain kinds of therapists' behaviors (empathic, option-enhancing behaviors) appear to induce or intensify positive or nondefensive attitudes toward therapy. Studies comparing relatively effective and ineffective therapists need to be completed so that we might further our understanding of how IPT-M serves to protect patients from a recurrence of illness and so that our procedures for selecting, training, and monitoring therapists might more effectively enhance their ability to consistently provide high-quality treatment across a range of patients. IPT provides a unique opportunity to study what we call "universal interpersonal change processes," or how work on improving interpersonal relationships can lead to longer wellness intervals (e.g., what kinds of therapist interventions inspire a patient to take responsibility for his or her relationships and for taking an active stance to interpersonal problem solving?).

Optimizing the Efficacy of IPT-M

Although one session per week for 12–20 weeks has become an industry standard for the "short-term" psychotherapy of depression, there is little empirical evidence to support this particular format of therapy. It may well be that a better outcome could be produced by having more frequent sessions early in treatment to accelerate the recovery process, with sessions spaced further apart as treatment proceeds. With respect to maintenance IPT, although monthly sessions showed a significant effect in extending the interval between depressive episodes, somewhat more frequent contact (e.g., every other week) may produce an even better outcome. A controlled trial testing this question in women with recurrent depression is currently under way.

Testing IPT in Other Patient Groups and Disorders

Currently, adaptations of IPT are being tested in other age groups (e.g., adolescents and the elderly), for other mood disorders (e.g., dysthymia and bipolar disorder), and for other life-threatening medical disorders (e.g., depressed HIV-positive patients). Another promising area in testing the generalizability of IPT is the application of IPT in oncology. Specifically, given empirical evidence that the principal psychosocial sequelae of breast cancer and its treatment are symptoms of depression and anxiety (see Moyer and Salovey 1996 for a review), testing an adaptation of IPT as a psychosocial intervention for women diagnosed with breast cancer appears to hold particular promise for improving quality of life and possibly extending survival time. The relative ease with which IPT could be adapted to this clinical population is another important consideration. Cancer itself is a stressful life event with a breadth and depth of interpersonal and social repercussions. Clearly the four IPT problem areas—grief, role transition, interpersonal disputes, and interpersonal deficits—have direct applicability in a condition marked by emotional distress (e.g., depression and anxiety), time constraints, and losses and disruptions in the social environment (e.g., employment) and relationships (e.g., loss of intimacy, emotional distancing, and closure). Thus another challenge for the future is the piloting of IPT adapted for distressed breast cancer patients and then testing its efficacy and effectiveness in this condition.

References

Bearden C, Lavelle NM, Buysse D, et al: Personality pathology and time to response in depressed patients treated with interpersonal psychotherapy (IPT). Journal of Personality Disorders 10:164–173, 1996

Bebbington PE, Brugha T, MacCarthy B, et al: The Camberwell Collaborative Depression Study, I: depressed probands: adversity and the form of depression. Br J Psychiatry 152:754–765, 1988

Bebbington PE, Der G, MacCarthy B, et al: Stress incubation and the onset of affective disorders. Br J Psychiatry 362:358–362, 1993

Bowlby J: The making and breaking of affectional bonds, I: aetiology and psychopathology in the light of attachment theory. Br J Psychiatry 130:201–210, 1977a

Bowlby J: The making and breaking of affectional bonds, II: some principles of psychotherapy. Br J Psychiatry 130:421–431, 1977b

Bowlby J: Attachment and Loss, Vol I: Attachment, 2nd Edition. New York, Basic Books, 1982

Brown GW, Harris TO: Social Origins of Depression: A Study of Psychiatric Disorder in Women. London, Tavistock, 1978

Brown GW, Harris TO: Life Events and Illness. New York, Guilford, 1989

Brown GW, Harris TO, Hepworth C: Life events and endogenous depression. Arch Gen Psychiatry 51:525–534, 1994

Buysse DJ, Kupfer DJ: Sleep disorders in depressive disorders, in Biology of Depressive Disorders, Part A: A Systems Perspective. Edited by Mann JJ, Kupfer DJ. New York, Plenum, 1993, pp 123–154

Crits-Christoph P, Mintz J: Implications of therapist effects for the design and analysis of comparative studies of psychotherapies. J Consult Clin Psychol 59:20–26, 1991

DiMascio A, Weissman MM, Prusoff BA, et al: Differential symptom reduction by drugs and psychotherapy in acute depression. Arch Gen Psychiatry 36:1450–1456, 1979

Elkin I, Shea MT, Watkins JT, et al: NIMH Treatment of Depression Collaborative Research Program, I: general effectiveness of treatments. Arch Gen Psychiatry 46:971–982, 1989

Frank E: Interpersonal psychotherapy as a maintenance treatment for patients with recurrent depression. Psychotherapy 28:259–266, 1991

Frank E, Kupfer DJ: Maintenance therapy in depression: in reply. Arch Gen Psychiatry 51:504–505, 1994

Frank E, Spanier CA: Interpersonal psychotherapy for depression: overview, clinical efficacy, and future directions. Clinical Psychology Science and Practice 2:349–369, 1995

Frank E, Kupfer DJ, Jacob M, et al: Personality features and response to acute treatment in recurrent depression. J Affective Disord 1:14–26, 1987

Frank E, Kupfer DJ, Perel JM, et al: Three-year outcomes for maintenance therapies in recurrent depression. Arch Gen Psychiatry 47:1093–1099, 1990

Frank E, Kupfer DJ, Wagner EF, et al: Efficacy of interpersonal psychotherapy as a maintenance treatment of recurrent depression: contributing factors. Arch Gen Psychiatry 48:1053–1059, 1991

Frank E, Kupfer DJ, Cornes C, et al: Maintenance interpersonal psychotherapy for recurrent depression, in New Applications of Interpersonal Psychotherapy. Edited by Klerman GL, Weissman MM. Washington, DC, American Psychiatric Press, 1993, pp 75–102

Frank E, Anderson B, Reynolds CF, et al: Life events and the research diagnostic criteria endogenous subtype: a confirmation of the distinction using the Bedford College methods. Arch Gen Psychiatry 51:519–524, 1994

Greenhouse JB, Stangl D, Bromberg J: An introduction to survival analysis: statistical methods for analysis of clinical trial data. J Consult Clin Psychol 57:536–544, 1989

Hamilton M: A rating scale for depression. J Neurol Neurosurg Psychiatry 23:56–62, 1960

Jacobson S, Deykin E, Prusoff B: Process and outcome of therapy with depressed women. Am J Orthopsychiatry 47:140–148, 1977

Klerman GL, DiMascio A, Weissman M, et al: Treatment of depression by drugs and psychotherapy. Am J Psychiatry 131:186–191, 1974

Klerman GL, Weissman MM, Rounsaville BJ, et al: Interpersonal Psychotherapy of Depression. New York, Basic Books, 1984

Kupfer DJ, Frank E, McEachran AB, et al: Delta sleep ratio: a biological correlate of early recurrence in unipolar affective disorder. Arch Gen Psychiatry 47:1100–1105, 1990

Kupfer DJ, Frank E, Perel JM, et al: Five-year outcome for maintenance therapies in recurrent depression. Arch Gen Psychiatry 49:769–773, 1992

Luborsky L, McLellan AT, Woody GE, et al: Therapist success and its determinants. Arch Gen Psychiatry 42:602–611, 1985

Lyubomirsky S, Nolen-Hoeksema S: Self-perpetuating properties of dysphoric rumination. J Pers Soc Psychol 65:339–349, 1993

Lyubomirsky S, Nolen-Hoeksema S: Effects of self-focused rumination on negative thinking and interpersonal problem-solving. J Pers Soc Psychol 69:176–190, 1995

Moyer A, Salovey P: Psychosocial sequelae of breast cancer and its treatment. Behav Med 16:110–125, 1996

O'Malley SS, Foley SH, Rounsaville BJ, et al: Therapist competence and patient outcome in interpersonal psychotherapy of depression. J Consult Clin Psychol 56:496–501, 1988

Pilkonis PA, Frank E: Personality pathology in recurrent depression: nature, prevalence, and relationship to treatment response. Am J Psychiatry 145:435–441, 1988

Prochaska JO, Norcross JC: Interpersonal Therapies. Systems of Psychotherapy: A Transtheoretical Analysis, 3rd Edition. Pacific Grove, CA, Brooks/Cole, 1994, pp 191–225

Raskin A, Schulterbrandt J, Reatig N, et al: Replication of factors of psychopathology in interview, ward behavior, and self-report ratings of hospitalized depressives. J Nerv Ment Dis 148:87–98, 1969

Rounsaville BJ, Chevron ES, Prusoff BA: The relation between specific and general dimensions of the psychotherapy process in interpersonal psychotherapy of depression. J Consult Clin Psychol 55:379–384, 1987

Singer JD, Willett JB: Quantitative methods in psychology. Modeling the days of our lives: using survival analysis when designing and analyzing longitudinal studies of duration and the timing of events. Psychol Bull 110:268–290, 1991

Spanier CA: The prevention of depression: protective mechanisms of maintenance interpersonal psychotherapy. Doctoral dissertation, University of Pittsburgh, 1997. Dissertation Abstracts International, University microfilms no. 9812397, 1997

Spanier CA, Frank E, McEachran AB, et al: The prophylaxis of depressive episodes in recurrent depression following discontinuation of drug therapy: integrating psychological and biological factors. Psychol Med 26:461–475, 1996

Stiles WB, Shapiro DA, Elliott R: Are all psychotherapies equivalent? Am Psychol 7:165–180, 1986

Sullivan HS: The Interpersonal Theory of Psychiatry. New York, WW Norton, 1953

Weissman MM, Markowitz JC: Interpersonal psychotherapy: current status. Arch Gen Psychiatry 51:599–606, 1994

Weissman MM, Klerman GL, Paykel ES, et al: Treatment effects on the social adjustment of depressed patients. Arch Gen Psychiatry 30:771–778, 1974

Chapter 4

Interpersonal Psychotherapy for Bulimia Nervosa

Christopher G. Fairburn, D.M., F.R.C.Psych.

Interpersonal psychotherapy (IPT) is a short-term focal psychotherapy in which the goal is to help patients identify and modify current interpersonal problems. It was developed in the late 1960s as a treatment for clinical depression, the premise being that since interpersonal difficulties contribute to the onset and maintenance of depression their resolution is likely to hasten recovery.

More recently IPT has been applied to other problems, including recurrent depression, bipolar disorder, substance abuse, marital problems, and eating disorders (Klerman and Weissman 1993; Weissman and Markowitz 1994). In addition, adaptations have been devised for adolescents (Mufson et al. 1993) and the elderly (Frank et al. 1993). In this chapter I focus on its application to bulimia nervosa.

The Status of IPT for Bulimia Nervosa

Two studies, both conducted by my group at Oxford, provide empirical support for the use of IPT to treat bulimia nervosa. In the first (Fairburn et al. 1986), a form of cognitive-behavioral

This chapter is adapted from Garner DM, Garfinkel PE (eds): *Handbook of Treatment for Eating Disorders*. New York, Guilford, 1997. Used with permission.

The research described in the chapter was supported by grants from the U.K. Medical Research Council (8008656 and 8921076) and the Wellcome Trust (13961). I hold a Wellcome Trust Principal Research Fellowship (046386).

therapy (CBT) designed specifically for treating bulimia nervosa (Fairburn 1981; Fairburn et al. 1993b) was compared with a short-term focal psychotherapy in which the emphasis was on identifying and modifying interpersonal problems accompanying the eating disorder rather than the eating disorder itself. This treatment was nondirective and noninterpretative in character. In its first stage, current interpersonal problems were identified from a detailed assessment of the patient's past and from an examination of the circumstances under which episodes of overeating tended to occur. In the second stage, these problems became the focus of treatment, with patients being encouraged to think about them in depth and consider possible ways of changing. In the final few sessions the focus shifted toward reviewing what had been learned in treatment and applying it to the future.

The results were striking (see Figure 4–1). Patients in both treatment conditions improved substantially, with the changes being maintained over a 12-month treatment-free follow-up period. Although some findings favored CBT, it was nevertheless clear that the focal interpersonal therapy had a major and sustained impact on the disorder.

The second Oxford study (Fairburn et al. 1991, 1993a) was designed to replicate and extend the findings of the first study using a larger sample size. Seventy-five patients were randomized to three treatments—CBT, behavior therapy (BT), and IPT. CBT was essentially the same treatment as that used in the first trial. BT was a dismantled version of CBT consisting solely of behavioral procedures directed at normalizing eating. IPT was chosen in place of the original interpersonal treatment since it was similar to it in style and focus while having the advantage of being better known and having a treatment manual available.

The findings at the end of treatment indicated that all three treatments had a substantial effect, with the results favoring CBT (Fairburn et al. 1991). However, the effects of the three treatments differed over time. Patients who received BT did not do well: indeed, over the 12-month treatment-free follow-up period, almost half of the patients either dropped out or had to be withdrawn on clinical grounds. The poor maintenance of change with

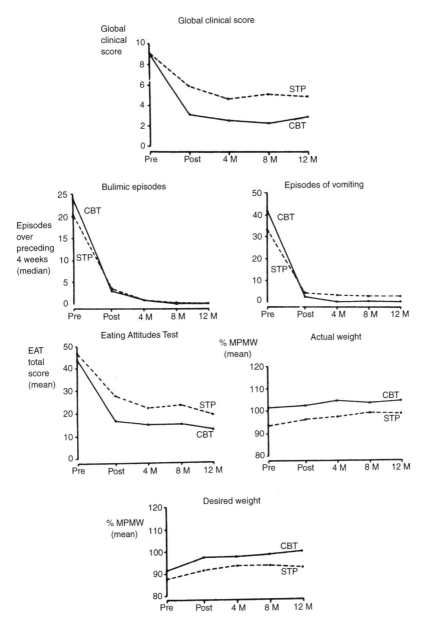

Figure 4–1. Changes in eating disorder psychopathology and weight following treatment with cognitive-behavioral therapy (CBT) or short-term focal psychotherapy (STP). MPMW, matched population mean weight; EAT, Eating Attitudes Test.

Source. Reprinted from Fairburn CG, Kirk J, O'Connor M, et al.: "A Comparison of Two Psychological Treatments for Bulimia Nervosa." *Behav Res Ther* 24:629–643, 1986. Used with permission from Elsevier Science.

BT is illustrated by the rapid decline in the proportion who met strict criteria for a good outcome (see Figure 4–2). This course of events contrasts sharply with that following CBT and IPT, where there was no tendency for the patients' states to deteriorate (Fairburn et al. 1993a). As can be seen in Figure 4–2, CBT achieved its effects rapidly, with almost all of the changes occurring during treatment itself, whereas with IPT the changes were slower to develop but continued during follow-up.

Recently the patients in these two trials have been reassessed, the average length of follow-up being 6 years (Fairburn et al.

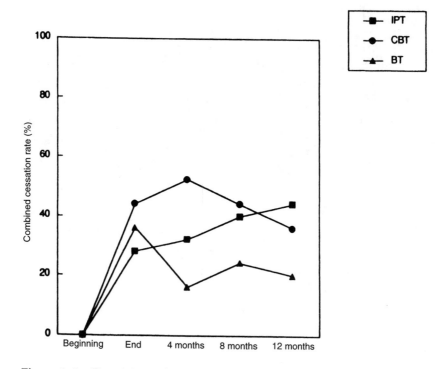

Figure 4–2. Proportions of patients who met strict criteria for a good outcome following cognitive-behavioral therapy (CBT), behavior therapy (BT), or interpersonal psychotherapy (IPT).
Source. Reprinted from Fairburn CG, Jones R, Peveler RC, et al.: "Psychotherapy and Bulimia Nervosa: The Longer-Term Effects of Interpersonal Psychotherapy, Behaviour Therapy, and Cognitive Behaviour Therapy." *Arch Gen Psychiatry* 50:419–428, 1993. Used with permission. Copyright 1993 American Medical Association.

1995). Perhaps surprisingly, given the length of follow-up and the fact that more than a third had received subsequent treatment (the proportion being the same across the three treatment groups), differential treatment effects were observed even after this long interval. Subjects who had received BT fared the worst: at follow-up 86% had a DSM-IV (American Psychiatric Association 1994) eating disorder compared with 37% and 28% of those who had received CBT or one of the two forms of focal interpersonal psychotherapy, respectively. These findings are similar to those at 12-month follow-up. They indicate that BT had an immediate but short-lived effect, with patients subsequently tending to relapse. In contrast, the majority of patients who received CBT or focal interpersonal psychotherapy did well, with the treatment effects observed at the 12-month follow-up evaluation being still present on average 6 years later.

Taken together, the findings of these two trials provide strong evidence that bulimia nervosa responds to psychological treatments that are not cognitive-behavioral in character. However, the studies do not imply that bulimia nervosa responds to any psychological intervention—far from it. The relative ineffectiveness of BT is testimony to this fact. Furthermore, it is common clinical experience that many patients with bulimia nervosa have received psychotherapy in the past with limited or only transitory benefit. What the findings of the two Oxford trials suggest is that short-term psychotherapies that focus on modifying current interpersonal problems are a promising alternative to CBT. IPT is the leading treatment of this kind.

The Practice of Interpersonal Psychotherapy for Bulimia Nervosa

IPT for bulimia nervosa (IPT-BN), as developed by the author and his colleagues at Oxford, closely resembles IPT for depression. Thus it is a noninterpretative, nondirective form of individual psychotherapy involving 15–20 50-minute sessions over 4–5 months. The treatment has three stages, each of which is described in the following. For further details about the practice of IPT, readers should consult the IPT manual (Klerman et al. 1984).

Stage 1

Stage 1 usually occupies three to four sessions. The goals are threefold:

1. To describe the rationale and nature of IPT.
2. To identify current interpersonal problems.
3. To choose which of the interpersonal problems should become the focus of the remainder of treatment.

Describing the Rationale and Nature of IPT

To help people break out of a self-perpetuating problem such a bulimia nervosa it is necessary to find out what is keeping it going and then address the maintaining factors in treatment. Interpersonal difficulties are common in patients with bulimia nervosa, although many have limited awareness of them because of the distracting influence of their preoccupation with thoughts about eating, shape, and weight. The interpersonal difficulties play an important role in maintaining the eating disorder through a number of mechanisms; for example, many binges are precipitated by interpersonal events and circumstances such as having an argument or feeling lonely. The therapist might explain this perspective as follows:

> The relevance of relationships to bulimia nervosa has been highlighted by the results of two recent treatment studies, which have shown that treatments that modify current interpersonal problems have a major beneficial effect that appears to be well maintained. IPT is the best substantiated of these treatments.

In IPT there is little emphasis on the patient's eating problem as such except during the assessment stage (stage 1). Instead, the focus is on the patient's interpersonal difficulties. This approach is taken because focusing on the eating disorder would tend to distract the patient and therapist from dealing with the interpersonal difficulties.

Patients are also forewarned that IPT has two distinct phases that are quite different in character. In the first, which occupies the first three or four sessions, the goal is to identify the interpersonal difficulties on which to focus. The therapist might say:

> This stage of treatment will involve a detailed review of your past and present relationships, and I will take the lead in asking you questions; it will end with us agreeing on the problem or problems that should be the focus of the remainder of treatment. Thereafter our sessions will change in style. You will become largely responsible for the content of the sessions, and I will take more of a backseat role. Gradually we will learn more about your interpersonal difficulties and ways of changing them. Your role will be not only to explore these difficulties in our treatment sessions but also to experiment with ways of changing. Doing so will shed further light on the nature of your problems and may lead to change.

It is important to stress the time-limited nature of the treatment. As performed in Oxford, IPT has a fixed number of sessions, usually 16, which are held at weekly intervals until near the end of treatment, when they are held every 2 weeks. Therefore, even at the outset it is possible to give the patient a good idea of when treatment is likely to end. That the treatment has a fixed number of sessions helps the therapist stress the importance of working hard at treatment:

> This is an opportunity to change—an opportunity to break out of what has been a long-standing problem. It is essential that you make the most of the opportunity by giving the treatment priority in your life. Not doing so is likely to limit the progress we can make.

Other ground rules also need to be explained. For example, in Oxford we say that sessions will always end on time (50 minutes after they are due to start), and it is the responsibility of both the therapist and patient to ensure that they start promptly. Exchanging telephone numbers in case of unforeseen problems is a good idea.

Identifying Current Interpersonal Problems

Three sources of information are used to identify current interpersonal problems.

---

1. A history is taken of the interpersonal context in which the eating problem developed and has been maintained. This history helps in identifying current interpersonal problems. It also highlights links between changes in the eating problem and the occurrence of interpersonal events, thereby stressing the importance of interpersonal factors. This aspect helps the patient to see the relevance of this form of treatment.

Four separate histories are taken starting from birth. The first is a history of the eating problem and how it has evolved. Key events and dates are recorded (e.g., the ages at which the patient first began to diet, binge, and purge). The timing of major changes in weight are noted, as is prior experience with treatment. The second history is of the patient's interpersonal functioning before and since the development of the eating problem. Relationships with family and peers are especially relevant here. The third history is of significant life events, many of which will already have been identified. The fourth history is of problems with self-esteem and depression. The history taking should culminate in the creation of a life chart in which separate columns are allocated to each domain. A typical life chart is shown in Table 4–1.

The patient should be encouraged to play an active role in the history taking and creation of the life chart. Looking through old diaries and photographs can be helpful, as can discussions with relatives and friends. The whole process usually takes two to three sessions.

2. An assessment is made of the quality of the patient's current interpersonal functioning. This assessment involves asking about the patient's social network. Inquiry should be made about family members, the patient's partner, confidants, friends, work contacts, and other acquaintances. The topics to be addressed include frequency of contact, positive and negative aspects of each relationship, mutual expectations, intimacy, and reciprocity.

3. The precipitants of bulimic episodes are identified. In each of the assessment sessions, the therapist asks whether there have been any binges (objective or subjective) and, if so, inquires about the circumstances preceding them. Since it is common for bulimic episodes to be precipitated by interpersonal events, they serve as markers of current interpersonal problems.

Choosing Which Problem Areas Should Become the Focus of Treatment

By the third or fourth session the nature of the patient's interpersonal difficulties should be clear. Usually they belong to one of the four standard problem areas recognized in the IPT manual: grief, interpersonal disputes, role transitions, or interpersonal deficits. (These problem areas are discussed later in the chapter.) The next step is for the patient and therapist to decide together which of the problem areas should become the focus of the remainder of treatment. When more than one problem is identified, progress is facilitated if the therapist suggests the order in which they should be tackled. Generally it is best if the simplest and most soluble of the problems is addressed first; for example, unresolved grief can often be tackled relatively quickly, in part because it does not generally require others to change. Tackling the most soluble problem first also has the advantage that progress on one front often leads to progress on others. The patient's morale and overall sense of competence are enhanced by making progress on a problem, and barriers to progress in other areas may be eroded or even removed altogether.

In some cases the interpersonal problems identified have no clear connection to the eating disorder. IPT appears to be just as useful in these cases, an observation that suggests that it operates at least in part through general mechanisms rather than simply by tackling the immediate precipitants of binges.

Stage 2

The second and third stages of the treatment are virtually identical to IPT for depression, as described in the IPT manual, al-

Table 4–1. Life chart for a person with bulimia nervosa

Age	Eating problem	Relationships	Events or circumstances	Depression or low self-esteem
13		No friends, called a snob	Change in school	
14	Begins to diet, rapid weight loss			
15	Meets criteria for anorexia nervosa			
	Starts to binge, weight begins to rise			Depressive symptoms develop
16	Starts to vomit, weight now back to previous level			Pronounced depressive symptoms
17	Regular binge eating and vomiting (meets criteria for bulimia nervosa)			

Age			
18	Eating disorder detected by psychiatrist Short-lived improvement in eating habits		Referred to psychiatrist for treatment of depression Receives antidepressants and psychotherapy	Short-lived improvement in depression
19	Transitory decrease in frequency of binge eating and vomiting, some weight loss	Spends much time with V. (girlfriend from school) Starts at college		
20		Starts seeing R. (boyfriend) Major argument with parents over vacation plans		
21				
22		Breakup of friendship with V., accused of being "aloof," "arrogant," and "dependent"	Seeks help from college doctor	Worsening of depressive symptoms

though in IPT-BN the patient is perhaps placed under greater pressure to change. Stage 2 generally involves about eight weekly sessions.

At the end of stage 1 the therapist reminds the patient that the treatment will now change in character:

> As we discussed at the outset, from this point on the nature of our sessions will change. Instead of me asking you questions, you will take the lead. Your task will be to focus on the problems we have identified and consider them in depth and from all possible angles. In this way you will come to a better understanding of them. A key part of this process is thinking about what changes are possible and how you could bring them about. You will need to consider all of the possible alternatives and their pros and cons. And it is important that you experiment with ways of changing, since by doing so you will not only get a better idea of the nature of the problems but may well be able to influence them as well.

The sessions from this point on are largely patient led. The therapist's job is to ensure that the patient remains focused on the identified problem areas, gains a better understanding of them, and attempts to change. After reminding the patient of the session number and how many remain, sessions are opened by a general inquiry such as "Where shall we start today?" Thereafter, the patient takes the lead.

The therapist is active but not directive. The patient is encouraged to explore the problem areas and consider ways of changing. Attempts to change then become the focus of subsequent sessions. The therapist helps the patient remain focused by ensuring that the subject matter is relevant and by providing clarification when needed. For example, a patient described helping her father remodel his house. This discussion was relevant since their relationship was one of the agreed problem areas. However, when she went on to discuss the nature of the adaptation, the therapist had to intervene since the interpersonal focus had been lost. Clarification takes the form of pointing out themes and inconsistencies, highlighting points that the patient might miss. For example, a patient had three problem areas that appeared quite distinct. The therapist made an important clarificatory intervention by pointing out that contributing to each problem was the patient's desire to avoid conflict at all cost. Clarification does not extend to making interpretations in which reference is made to a theoretical view on the disorder and its treatment. Throughout, the focus remains on the present.

The therapist should ensure that the patient remains aware of the task at hand. At the end of each session it is our practice at Oxford to provide a brief résumé in which the therapist summarizes what has been covered. In addition, at intervals during stage 2, we review progress by considering each of the problem areas and assessing what has been achieved and what remains to be done.

In the Oxford version of the treatment the need to change is stressed at regular intervals. It is important to note that this emphasis constitutes general encouragement to change rather than pressure to take a specific course of action. As illustrated later, the therapist is active in supporting and reinforcing attempts to change but is not directive in the sense of making specific recommendations. Formal problem solving, as used in CBT treatments, is not employed, although the therapist helps patients to consider the various options available to them. Behavioral procedures are used rarely. Exceptions include the reenacting of key exchanges to get a clearer idea of what was said and the role-playing of important future exchanges. For example, a patient was about to face a job interview after having been off work for more than a year. Having encouraged her to consider how she would account for the period of unemployment, the therapist helped the patient to rehearse her response at the interview through the use of role-playing.

Rarely is reference made to the therapist-patient relationship since doing so can complicate and undermine IPT. An exception is when treating patients with interpersonal deficits whose social network is so impoverished that one of the few relationships available for examination is that between the therapist and patient. Reference to the therapist-patient relationship can also be useful with patients who would be helped by feedback about how they come across to others. This issue is illustrated later in the chapter.

Interestingly, most patients make few, if any, references to their eating disorder. If they do, our practice has been to shift the focus away from the eating problem and onto its interpersonal context. Detailed discussion of the eating disorder and its symptomatic management are not part of IPT-BN as evaluated to date (see this chapter's final section).

Stage 3

The third stage of treatment comprises the final three or four sessions. These sessions, which may be held at 2-week intervals, address two related goals. The first is to ensure that the changes that have been made during treatment continue following discharge, and the second is to minimize the risk of relapse.

Unlike the transition between stages 1 and 2, there is no sharp change in style between stages 2 and 3. Instead, the sessions continue much as before, with the addition of a review of treatment in which what has been achieved and what has not are considered. When progress on a particular problem area is being discussed, the therapist should help the patient project forward: "As you know, we only have three more sessions to go. What do you envisage happening regarding . . . over the coming months? How can you make sure that you build on what you have achieved so far?" By this point it should be clear what changes are likely to be made and what changes may not take place. The therapist should ensure that the patient has realistic expectations. For example, the therapist might say, "Given what has emerged during treatment, it seems unlikely that . . . will start to behave differently in the foreseeable future. If this is the case, what do you think you should do?" The therapist should also help the patient predict areas of future difficulty.

It is not uncommon for patients at this stage in treatment to make reference to their eating problem. Unless it is so troublesome as to make the ending of treatment impossible, our practice is to remind patients that the evidence suggests that it often takes months for the full benefits of IPT to be felt (as illustrated in Figure 4–2) (Fairburn et al. 1993a). We point out to patients tempted to start further treatment that in our opinion they might best delay doing so, since in this way they will be able to see whether there is continuing improvement and, if so, attribute it to the changes that they have already set in motion, something they would be unable to do were they to undergo further treatment. However, the patients are also told that their eating problem is likely to remain an Achilles' heel in the sense that it may recur at future times of difficulty. We encourage patients to view any return of symptoms as a useful early warning signal that requires them to review what is happening in their lives and perhaps take some action.

It is unusual for patients receiving IPT to have difficulty accepting the ending of treatment because it is made clear at the outset that treatment is time limited and at the beginning of each session they are reminded of the number of sessions remaining. Nevertheless therapists should always ask patients how they feel about the ending of treatment, not least because this question provides an opportunity to emphasize what has been achieved and to stress patients' competence at dealing with future areas of difficulty.

The Four Problem Areas

Grief.   Our experience suggests that problems with grief are not common among patients with bulimia nervosa. They were judged to be present among 12% of the patients in our trial. As mentioned earlier, they often resolve comparatively quickly, and it is therefore worth addressing them first. The goal is to help patients face the loss, assess exactly what has been lost, and start to move on (Klerman et al. 1984).

Interpersonal role disputes.   Interpersonal disputes were present in 64% of the patients in our trial. Such disputes may be with any figure of importance in the patients' lives, including their partners, parents, children, friends, and employers. The aim of treatment is to help clarify the nature of the dispute, consider the possibilities for change on both sides, and then actively explore them. The outcome may be a renegotiation of the relationship or its dissolution.

Role transitions.   Problems with role transitions are common in this patient group. Not surprisingly, given their age, these difficulties often involve establishing independence from their parents. The goal of treatment is to help the patient abandon the old role and adopt a new one. Treatment involves exploring exactly what the new role involves and how it can be mastered. Associated role disputes often need to be addressed at the same time.

Problems with role transitions are not confined to the difficulties of late adolescence and early adulthood. They also include problems coping with other life changes such as leaving college, changing jobs, getting married, and becoming a parent. They were judged to be present among 36% of the patients in our trial.

Interpersonal deficits.   Interpersonal deficits are present when the patient gives a long history of difficulty initiating or maintaining intimate relationships. Some degree of social isolation is common in bulimia nervosa and needs to be addressed, but longstanding interpersonal deficits are much less common. They were present in just 16% of the patients in our trial. This low prevalence is fortunate since such patients are difficult to help and many have an avoidant or schizoid personality disorder as defined in DSM-IV.

An Illustrative Case History

The patient was a 22-year-old university student studying physics. She was referred by her primary care physician for the treatment of an "intractable eating problem." Assessment indicated that she had the purging type of bulimia nervosa. In addition, she met criteria for major depressive disorder. Both disorders had been present since she was 16 years of age.

She complained of being "unable to stop eating" and denied having any other problems. She had recurrent objective bulimic episodes, many of which involved the consumption of very large amounts of food. These episodes, which occurred at least daily, were followed by compensatory self-induced vomiting. She also took large quantities of laxatives several times a week. Between the bulimic episodes she dieted to an extreme degree, her goal being to eat less than 1,200 calories daily. She was vigilant about her appearance and weighed herself at least twice daily. She was 5 foot 7 inches tall and 137 pounds in weight (body mass index = 22).

Stage 1

The therapist, who had not been involved in the patient's assessment, introduced himself. He asked about the processes that had led to her referral. She explained that 2 months earlier she had sought help from her primary care physician. The physician had provided simple counseling and advice, but it had proved unhelpful. Her doctor had therefore suggested that specialist help was needed, especially since the problem was long-standing and the patient had not benefited from treatment in the past.

The therapist described the nature and rationale of IPT (as outlined earlier). It was agreed that treatment would involve 16 weekly sessions. The likely date of the final session was identified.

The remainder of the first session and the next three sessions were devoted to identification of current interpersonal problems.

Identifying Current Interpersonal Problems

1. The interpersonal history.   The patient's problems with eating began when she was 14 years of age, shortly after she changed schools. She started to diet and over 6 months lost more than 20 pounds. Although the diagnosis was not made at the time, she met diagnostic criteria for anorexia nervosa. At the age of 15, her control over eating began to break down and her weight started to increase. At first her binges were small, but once she started to vomit as well they increased in size to become true DSM-IV binges (Fairburn and Wilson 1993). By the time she was 16 (the timing was relatively easy to locate since it could be related to specific school grades), her current eating pattern was established and her weight had increased to its present level.

In her last year at school, when she was 18, she was referred to a local psychiatrist for the treatment of depression. The psychiatrist detected the eating disorder, and the patient was treated with antidepressant drugs and a form of dynamic psychotherapy. This treatment resulted in a slight improvement in mood and eating habits, but the benefits were short-lived.

Over the subsequent 4 years her binge eating and vomiting continued unchanged. There was a slight improvement on coming up to Oxford, but she continued to eat little outside of her binges and for a while lost weight. The only other change was that 4 months before being referred for treatment she had begun to misuse laxatives.

From her personal history it emerged that she was an only child who was brought up in a city west of Oxford. Her father was a lawyer and her mother a teacher. Both were very involved in their work. The parents had liberal values, although there was a clear stated expectation that the patient would "do well" and go to Oxford, as they themselves had done. Neither parent showed the patient much affection during her childhood but for different reasons. Her father seemed uncomfortable expressing his feelings, but she felt sure that he was fond of her. In contrast, she found her mother "distant," "cold," and rivalrous. Her relationship with her parents had deteriorated over the previous summer when they had a protracted argument over how she was to spend the vacation. She wanted to travel abroad with a girlfriend, but her parents forbade it, saying that she was too young, it was not safe, and she ought to be using the time more productively.

The first event of note in her history was the change in school when she was 13 years of age. Having been at an ordinary local school, she was transferred to an avant-garde school favored by her parents. This school had little structure or discipline, and among the pupils a casual attitude toward work was de rigueur. She did not fit in since she enjoyed schoolwork, something that was strongly reinforced by her parents. She was rejected by the other children, who accused her of being a snob, possibly because of her parents' professional backgrounds and her accent. She had no friends or confidants. It was at this time that she began to diet. She spent 5 unhappy years at this school. Matters improved slightly in the last 2 years when she was taught with others planning to go on to university.

She came up to Oxford with one other person from her school. During their first 2 years they spent a great deal of time together. However, her friend became cooler at the beginning of the third year, and in the second term they had a major argument in which her friend described her as "dependent," "aloof," and "arrogant." Since then they had seen little of each other. This argument, and the considerable upset it caused, immediately preceded the start of the patient's laxative misuse.

Her problems with depression and low self-esteem tracked the state of her eating problem. They began shortly after she transferred to the avant-garde school and had persisted ever since. They had been particularly bad since the breakup of the relationship with her girlfriend. She thought that it was the feelings of depression and loneliness that had led her to seek help.

2. Current relationships. The loss of the relationship with the patient's girlfriend had been a great blow since she was her only confidant. The patient had a boyfriend, but they were not close. They had been going out for almost 2 years, but the relationship simply involved seeing each other on weekends and going to parties. The relationship had an aggressive side to it in that her boyfriend was offensive and rather uninvolved. On the other hand, she said that the relationship suited her since it was "not too bothersome."

She had no friends but did have a circle of people with whom she played darts in the college bar. She knew their names and what subjects they studied but little else.

3. Precipitants of bulimic episodes. Most of the patient's binges seemed to be habitual rather than triggered by specific events. She invariably overate in the afternoon and sometimes did so in the morning. Unlike many for patients with bulimia nervosa, she rarely overate in the evening. No specific triggers emerged other than the unstructured time and feelings of loneliness that characterized her afternoons.

Choosing Which Problem Areas Should Become the Focus of Treatment

Between the third and fourth sessions the therapist asked the patient to create a life chart summarizing her interpersonal history. An adaptation of this life chart is shown in Table 4–1. Clear links between her eating problem and the occurrence of interpersonal events were evident. On the basis of this information and that gathered from the assessment of her social network and the precipitants of her binges, the therapist proposed that focusing on the following three areas would be worthwhile:

1. *The difficulty with her parents.* This issue was presented as a role transition problem rather than as an interpersonal dispute. She was being treated as a child.
2. *The difficulties with her boyfriend.* The therapist suggested that there was an interpersonal dispute between her and her boyfriend since, contrary to her claims, it was likely that they had differing expectations of each other.
3. *Social isolation.* The therapist pointed out that her social network did not include any friends or confidants. The therapist did not class the problem as an interpersonal deficit (as defined earlier) since it appeared that she had the ability to form intimate relationships. Instead, he wondered whether there might be a social skills problem that acted as a barrier to the forming of relationships. The accusations of her being a "snob" and "arrogant" seemed relevant and worth exploring.

The patient accepted that exploring the first and third problem areas would be valuable. It was obvious that something had to be done about her relationship with her parents, and over the previous few months she had become increasingly aware of her social isolation. However, she did not regard the relationship with her boyfriend as a problem and so it was decided to put that issue aside.

The fifth session ended with the therapist reminding the patient that the sessions would now change in style.

Stage 2

The sixth session coincided with the end of term and the start of the long summer vacation. After the previous summer's argument with her parents, the patient had no specific plans about how to spend the 8 weeks other than she expected to be based at home. The therapist suggested that she ought to give treatment priority since this would maximize the chances of success. He also suggested that the patient being at home might make it easier to deal with the first of the agreed-upon problem areas, her relationship with her parents.

The patient talked about her concern that treatment was becoming too intrusive. She did not like dwelling on herself: "Life is bad enough without having to think about it the whole time." The therapist commented that one has to face up to problems in order to overcome them and that some degree of introspection is necessary to bring about change.

One topic dominated the seventh session. On arriving home the patient had decided to tell her parents about the eating problem, the first time she had mentioned it to them. Her parents reacted differently. Her father seemed genuinely shocked and at a loss as to what to say. Her mother said that she had known all along. Neither parent raised the subject again during the entire week. The patient was angry and upset at their lack of reaction. She had divulged a major problem, and her parents had barely responded. The patient then went on to describe her need to be perfect. She felt that she had been "infected" by her parents' drive to succeed and that this drive had made her "obsessed with performance." She had to succeed at everything she did. It was therefore highly significant for her to admit to her parents that she had an eating problem. Their lack of response was very hurtful. The therapist suggested that her parents' behavior reinforced the need for treatment to focus on her relationship with them. The patient agreed.

The patient was somewhat hostile in the next session. She said that she felt worse than when she had started treatment and disliked the lack of guidance. The therapist restated the rationale behind IPT and reason for not focusing on her eating. The patient then went on to discuss her parents' response to her admission that she had an eating problem. She said that her father seemed to be avoiding her. He was spending even more time than usual working in his study, and her mother was busying herself with preparations for the end of the school term. The patient felt angry and rejected.

Between the eighth and ninth sessions the patient raised with her parents the issue of their apparent indifference to her revelation. Both said that they wanted to help but were unsure how to do so. At a loss about what action to take, her father started to make awkward and inappropriate comments about what she ate. Her mother bought a number of self-help books on eating problems and left them on her bed, saying "these should help." The patient started to feel more angry than rejected and reported that her eating was awful. The therapist said that this was understandable given the tension at home.

The 10th session opened with the patient saying that she had been thinking about her relationship with her parents and felt that it was worth distinguishing between her parents' rights and their expectations. She thought that they had a right to expect her to make the most of her time at Oxford. It was also reasonable for them to expect her to fit into the home routine when she was with them during the vacation. On the other hand, given her age and circumstances, she thought it was inappropriate for them to expect her to be an outstanding academic and not reasonable for them to dictate what she did during the vacation. The therapist said that he thought that the distinction between rights and expectations seemed useful. He stressed the need to change, since this change might yield useful information.

At the 11th session the patient was more cheerful than she had been up to this point. She reported that the previous evening she had confronted her parents with their controlling behavior, their inappropriate expectations, and their apparent need for her to be perfect and trouble free. She told them that they needed to forge a new relationship since she was no longer going to accept the old one. She said that she would continue to work hard at Oxford and would obey reasonable house rules when at home, but in other respects she planned to follow her own priorities. Her parents responded by saying that they would think about what she had said. The therapist was strongly supportive of the patient.

Between the 11th and 12th sessions the patient returned to Oxford. The aftermath of the confrontation with her parents had been disappointing. They had simply carried on with their busy lives, not mentioning the subject at all. She had therefore decided to spend the remaining week or so of the vacation in Oxford. The therapist reinforced this decision, saying that it demonstrated to her parents her determination to redefine her relationship with them. It also fit in well with the stage she had reached in treatment. Although she had made considerable progress with respect to her parents, her social isolation had not been addressed. The therapist also suggested that it might be worth reconsidering her relationship with her boyfriend. The patient said that before the next session she would set aside time to think about these matters.

The 13th session opened with the patient saying that she had decided to break off her relationship with her boyfriend since it was basically unhealthy. Indeed, she announced that she had telephoned him to say that she did not intend to see him again. The therapist expressed concern at the abrupt termination of the relationship. The patient retorted that just as her relationship with her parents had needed attention so did her relationship with her boyfriend, but in this case there was little to be gained by continuing it. She thought that his aggression and offhand behavior were probably his way of coping with the fact that he felt threatened by her. She said that she wanted to establish a relationship with someone sufficiently secure to not be intimidated by her.

The therapist suggested that maybe many people found her intimidating and that this issue could be the basis of the accusations of her being arrogant and a snob. Since the patient seemed skeptical at this proposal, the therapist took the unusual step for IPT (see earlier) of commenting on his own experience of the patient, saying that he could see how people might find her threatening. He said that certain aspects of her behavior contributed to this impression. For example, her gait was striking in that she walked very fast and upright, rather like a model on a catwalk, and her speech was unusually rapid and fluent. As a result she had a self-confident air that might keep people at a distance. The therapist said that he suspected that a marked contrast existed between how he knew she felt about herself and her circumstances and how she was perceived by others.

The patient was taken aback by this intervention and started to cry. She began to talk about her loneliness. She also said that she had recently realized that she never admitted to having any problems. Although acquaintances at college would talk about their difficulties with work, boyfriends, and so forth, all she talked about were her achievements. She felt that she had learned this style of communicating from her parents, who only wanted to know about her accomplishments. She thought that it kept people at a distance and meant that she did not receive support from others. The therapist encouraged her to think more about this matter since he thought it was likely to contribute to her social isolation, the one problem that had not been addressed so far. He asked her to think about ways that she might be able to change.

Stage 3

The 14th session was dominated by further discussion of how the patient was perceived by others. She was convinced that this was a fundamental problem that had to be addressed and had decided to make two changes. First, she planned to be more open with others and to discuss any difficulties that she was having. Second, she thought that she would take up a sport. At school she had been dismissive of peers who were interested in sports, a view shared by her parents, but recently her attitude had changed and she felt envious of them. She thought that taking up a new sport would be a good way of getting to know a new circle of people and had decided to learn to play squash. The therapist supported these changes. Near the end of the session the therapist reminded her that there were just two more sessions remaining. She said that she was aware of the impending end of treatment and was worried since she felt that she was only just beginning to change. The therapist said that he thought that she had turned a corner and that he was confident that she would be able to build on what she had achieved.

The 15th session was much like the 14th. The patient reported that she was now spending more time with her fellow students. She was making a point of listening to their problems with work and discussing her own. She had told two students of her difficulties with eating, both of whom seemed amazed. She had also played squash on three occasions and was enjoying it.

The therapist used the last third of this session to review what had been achieved in treatment. The therapist and patient agreed that the difficulty with her parents had been addressed, although the extent to which her parents had changed was not clear. Fortuitously, her parents had contacted her earlier in the week saying that they would like to visit, which provided an opportunity for her to reassess her relationship with them. The second area of difficulty, the relationship with her boyfriend, had also been addressed, although only by eliminating it. Once again, the therapist expressed misgivings over the appropriateness of this solution, but the patient insisted that she had followed the right course of action. The therapist asked about future relationships with boyfriends and any problems she envisaged forming or maintaining them. The patient simply said that she would prefer no relationship over one with the wrong person. Finally, the therapist mentioned the third problem area, social isolation. It was agreed that definite progress was being made on this front.

At the final session the patient reported that the visit of her parents had gone well. They appeared interested in seeing her and had expressed concern about her overall well-being. The patient had enjoyed their visit and was looking forward to the

Christmas vacation. She thought that they seemed relieved that she was now doing things her way: it was as if a burden had been taken from them. In other respects there was little to report. She now had several friends in college whom she was seeing regularly, and her work was going well.

The therapist asked about her eating and mood. The patient seemed almost surprised at the question. She said that her eating had been awful over the summer but since being back in Oxford had improved greatly. She had not binged or vomited for 3 weeks—indeed, she had not given the problem much thought. She said that she also felt much better about herself and was no longer depressed in mood. The therapist told her that continuing improvement was likely. He also reminded her that binge eating serves as a marker of other difficulties and that it might recur at times of stress. Therefore, should there be a resurgence of the eating problem, she should take stock of her current situation.

Further Progress

Although no formal plans were made to follow up with the patient, she was contacted approximately 6 and 12 months after completing treatment. As predicted, her eating problem had continued to improve. At the 12-month follow-up she had no residual eating disorder psychopathology—she was not binge eating, vomiting, or misusing laxatives, and her scores on the Eating Disorder Examination subscales (Fairburn and Cooper 1993) were in the normal range. Socially, she had also made great strides. She had several close girlfriends, two of whom she had vacationed with in the summer. She also felt that she was more popular in college. Her relationship with her parents was much better than it had been; they now enjoyed each other's company. She had no boyfriend.

How Does IPT-BN Work?

Neither of the Oxford studies was designed to investigate how focal interpersonal psychotherapies work. The fact that IPT and

---

CBT are so different in practice makes it likely that, at least to some extent, they have their own particular modes of action. Our finding that IPT took longer than CBT to achieve its full effect supports this view (Fairburn et al. 1993a), although another possibility is that it operates through the same mechanisms as CBT but not as efficiently.

Our clinical observations as therapists may shed light on the mechanisms of action of IPT. We observed repeated instances of patients making major positive changes in their relationships, particularly with respect to parents, partners, peers, and employers. Often these changes set in motion other positive events, many of which were still evolving at the end of treatment. It seemed as if successful IPT might operate by bringing about fresh-start events (Brown et al. 1988). Although the precise relationship between interpersonal changes and alterations in eating disorder symptoms was not studied, and could not be assessed by the therapists since they were not aware of the state of the patients' eating problems, it is possible to see how improved interpersonal functioning could have a beneficial effect. At least four processes might operate:

1. The patients' realization that they are able to bring about changes in what have often been entrenched interpersonal problems might lead them to feel more capable of changing other aspects of their lives including their eating problems.
2. The improvement in mood and self-esteem might result in a decrease in the severity of the patients' concerns about appearance and weight, thereby reducing their tendency to diet and in turn their vulnerability to binge.
3. The increase in the patients' social activity might decrease the amount of unstructured time, thereby reducing their vulnerability to binge.
4. The reduction in the frequency and severity of interpersonal stressors might lead directly to a decrease in the frequency of binge eating.

Through the operation of processes of this type, it is not difficult to see how the eating disorder could be progressively eroded. It is also easy to see how the expression of the full effects of IPT might take longer than that of CBT, since CBT probably operates directly on the disturbed eating habits and attitudes whereas these changes may be secondary with IPT. However, the effects of IPT cannot be exclusively the product of changes in interpersonal functioning since some change occurs almost immediately.

Indications and Future Directions

In contrast to the substantial body of evidence supporting CBT as a treatment for bulimia nervosa (Fairburn et al. 1992; Wilson and Fairburn 1998), the evidence supporting IPT is much more modest. It cannot therefore be recommended as a first-line treatment. In my opinion, it is best viewed as a promising alternative to CBT. IPT should probably be reserved for patients who either fail to respond to CBT or who will not accept it. For example, we have had some success using IPT with patients who have both bulimia nervosa and insulin-dependent diabetes mellitus, a patient group that can be difficult to engage in CBT (Peveler and Fairburn 1992).

There is a clear need for more research on the use of IPT to treat bulimia nervosa. Nearing completion is a two-center trial (at Stanford and Columbia) in which the Oxford comparison of CBT and IPT is being repeated using the same treatment manuals and similar assessment measures. This study is designed to determine whether the original findings can be replicated. In addition, its large sample size will allow other important questions to be addressed. For example, an issue of considerable interest is whether the same types of patients benefit from the two treatments or whether there are mode-specific predictors of response. If different patient characteristics are found to predict response to CBT and IPT, this finding might allow the matching of patients to treatments, thereby improving overall outcome.

In addition to the necessity of substantiating the effectiveness of IPT, there is also a need to improve the treatment. Its cost-effectiveness might be enhanced by administering it in a group format. Work by Wilfley and colleagues (1993) with obese patients who binge eat suggests that this approach might be possible. The effectiveness of the treatment might be enhanced by adding techniques from CBT directed at the disturbed eating habits and attitudes. Indeed, it would seem logical to amalgamate IPT and CBT so that both the eating disorder and accompanying interpersonal problems are both directly addressed in a single treatment. Unfortunately this combination is not possible since the styles of the two treatments are so different as to make them immiscible. Instead, I and my colleagues have been experimenting with the combination of IPT and the cognitive-behavioral self-help book *Overcoming Binge Eating* (Fairburn 1995). Patients receive IPT exactly as described in this chapter while at the same time following the self-help program with the encouragement of the therapist. This combination seems to work well.

References

American Psychiatric Association: Diagnostic and Statistical Manual of Mental Disorders, 4th Edition. Washington, DC, American Psychiatric Association, 1994

Brown GW, Adler Z, Bifulco A: Life events, difficulties, and recovery from chronic depression. Br J Psychiatry 152:487–498, 1988

Fairburn CG: A cognitive behavioural approach to the management of bulimia. Psychol Med 11:707–711, 1981

Fairburn CG: Overcoming Binge Eating. New York, Guilford, 1995

Fairburn CG, Cooper Z: The Eating Disorder Examination, 12th Edition, in Binge Eating: Nature, Assessment, and Treatment. Edited by Fairburn CG, Wilson GT. New York, Guilford, 1993, pp 317–360

Fairburn CG, Wilson GT: Binge eating: definition and classification, in Binge Eating: Nature, Assessment, and Treatment. Edited by Fairburn CG, Wilson GT. New York, Guilford, 1993, pp 3–14

Fairburn CG, Kirk J, O'Connor M, et al: A comparison of two psychological treatments for bulimia nervosa. Behav Res Ther 24:629–643, 1986

Fairburn CG, Jones R, Peveler RC, et al: Three psychological treatments for bulimia nervosa: a comparative trial. Arch Gen Psychiatry 48:463–469, 1991

Fairburn CG, Agras WS, Wilson GT: The research on the treatment of bulimia nervosa: practical and theoretical implications, in The Biology of Feast and Famine: Relevance to Eating Disorders. Edited by Kennedy SH. San Diego, CA, Academic Press, 1992, pp 317–340

Fairburn CG, Jones R, Peveler RC, et al: Psychotherapy and bulimia nervosa: the longer-term effects of interpersonal psychotherapy, behaviour therapy, and cognitive behaviour therapy. Arch Gen Psychiatry 50:419–428, 1993a

Fairburn CG, Marcus MD, Wilson GT: Cognitive-behavioral therapy for binge eating and bulimia nervosa: a comprehensive treatment manual, in Binge Eating: Nature, Assessment, and Treatment. Edited by Fairburn CG, Wilson GT. New York, Guilford, 1993b, pp 361–404

Fairburn CG, Norman PA, Welch SL, et al: A prospective study of outcome in bulimia nervosa and the long-term effects of three psychological treatments. Arch Gen Psychiatry 52:304–312, 1995

Frank E, Frank N, Cornes C, et al: Interpersonal psychotherapy in the treatment of late-life depression, in New Applications of Interpersonal Therapy. Edited by Klerman GL, Weissman MM. Washington, DC, American Psychiatric Press, 1993, pp 167–198

Klerman GL, Weissman MM: New Applications of Interpersonal Psychotherapy. Washington, DC, American Psychiatric Press, 1993

Klerman GL, Weissman MM, Rounsaville BJ, et al: Interpersonal Psychotherapy of Depression. New York, Basic Books, 1984

Mufson L, Moreau D, Weissman MM, et al: Interpersonal Psychotherapy for Depressed Adolescents. New York, Guilford, 1993

Peveler RC, Fairburn CG: The treatment of bulimia nervosa in patients with diabetes mellitus. International Journal of Eating Disorders 11:45–53, 1992

Weissman MM, Markowitz JC: Interpersonal psychotherapy: current status. Arch Gen Psychiatry 51:599–606, 1994

Wilfley DE, Agras WS, Telch CF, et al: Group cognitive-behavioral therapy and group interpersonal psychotherapy for the nonpurging bulimic individual: a controlled comparison. J Consult Clin Psychol 61:296–305, 1993

Wilson GT, Fairburn CG: Treatments for eating disorders, in A Guide to Treatments That Work. Edited by Nathan PE, Gomai JM. New York, Oxford University Press, 1998, pp 501–530

Chapter 5

Interpersonal Psychotherapy for the Treatment of Depression in HIV-Positive Men and Women

Holly A. Swartz, M.D., and John C. Markowitz, M.D.

Psychotherapy, a mainstay of psychiatric treatment for a wide range of disorders and populations, is highly regarded by the profession yet relatively untested in controlled research settings. Historically, the discipline has relied on anecdotal case material and clinical impressions to validate the utility of treatment rather than on controlled outcome data (Lambert and Bergin 1994). To date, the evaluation of psychotherapy for the treatment of patients with the human immunodeficiency virus (HIV) also relies principally on anecdotal experience. The few extant controlled treatment studies are described in this chapter. The only psychotherapeutic modality to demonstrate a statistically significant advantage over another is interpersonal psychotherapy (IPT) (Markowitz et al. 1995). In this chapter we discuss the relationship between depression and HIV, describe the adaptation of IPT for the treatment of depression in HIV-positive individuals, and review the data demonstrating its efficacy in this population.

Depression and HIV

Weiner (1996) and others have wondered whether depression is an inevitable sequela of HIV infection. After all, this life-threatening illness strikes, in the prime of life, individuals whose only "fault" (used advisedly) may have been engaging in sexual intercourse, requiring a blood transfusion, or struggling with an addiction. Although advances in medical treatments have greatly increased patients' quality and duration of life, a cure eludes us. Both colleagues and laypersons have been wont to say, "If I had AIDS, I would be depressed, too."

Case Example

Mr. A, a 47-year-old Hispanic gay man who had known he was HIV-positive for 3 years, was referred for evaluation by his internist. Mr. A had been feeling well until he contracted Pneumocystis carinii pneumonia (PCP) 6 months before. He never fully recovered from the episode, experiencing persistent, unexplained weight loss, frequent episodes of crying, and difficulty concentrating that the internist felt was unrelated to the PCP. Mr. A had moved to New York City 20 years before, during the halcyon days of the gay community, from a small, Catholic, homophobic town in rural Chile. A saxophone player, Mr. A fondly remembers befriending other gay artists and socializing with a carefree abandon unknown to him in South America. He enjoyed the easy sexual exchanges and "non-stop partying" of those days.

As the acquired immunodeficiency syndrome (AIDS) epidemic advanced, his world crumbled. Literally hundreds of friends and acquaintances succumbed over just a few years. Mr. A reported, "I sometimes had trouble squeezing in a lunch date between funeral gigs." He enjoyed regular employment and the reputation of musical talent and remained seronegative until 3 years before evaluation. Mr. A stated, "You would think I would have been happy, but the world as I knew it had come to an end." Mr. A became involved in his first long-term relationship with 25-year-old, HIV-positive Fredo 5 years before seroconverting: "Fredo and I took a chance. We had a good time, but now I'm paying for it." Mr. A tolerated the stressors provoked by both the epidemic and his own serostatus without becoming depressed until he developed PCP. Although he spent only 4 days in the hospital, the pneumonia left residual scarring that significantly compromised his ability to play his wind instrument. He faced the prospect of being unable to return to work: "This disease took my friends, my fun, and my future. But now it's got my music, and that's one thing I can't live without."

As clinicians and human beings, we may have strong reactions to stories like Mr. A's and act on emotion rather than rational thinking. We may feel sorry for him, decide that his depression is "normal," and then assume treatment is hopeless. Mr. A, too, may assume that his depression is expected or that its symptoms are HIV related and accordingly avoid seeking treatment. Alternately, we may err on the side of overtreating, feeling that we are withholding support if we offer a briefer treatment instead of an open-ended one. The potent, emotional responses evoked by HIV may lead us astray: although empathy is invaluable in a clinical setting, intuitive hunches can be wrong; in the case of HIV, our assumptions frequently have been.

Despite predictions of rampant mood disorders in this population, researchers have found that rates of depression among HIV-positive subjects, although greater than rates in the general population, are similar to those in any medically ill population (Atkinson et al. 1988). Summarizing the American literature, Markowitz et al. (1994) reported that rates of current depressive disorders are estimated to be between 4% and 16% among HIV-positive, non-drug-using subjects. They noted several reports of substantially elevated lifetime rates of depression in HIV-positive populations and the finding that 78% of a depressed group of HIV-positive individuals seeking treatment had histories of depression before seroconversion (Rabkin et al. 1991).

Other studies report that while HIV does not increase the risk for current mood disorders per se, groups at high risk for HIV may, for unrelated reasons, experience an increased risk for depression. Perkins et al. (1994) studied 98 asymptomatic HIV-infected and 71 uninfected homosexual men. Although rates of lifetime (29% and 45%, respectively) and current (8% and 3%) major depression did not differ significantly between the groups, the prevalence of mood disorders in the entire sample was greater than rates in the general population, leading the authors to speculate that homosexual men may be at high risk for depression. Lipsitz et al. (1994) studied 124 HIV-positive and 99 HIV-negative intravenous drug users and found high rates of current depression (26%) in both groups, suggesting that, for a drug-using population, intravenous drug use may be more important than HIV status in determining risk for depression. Judd and Mijch (1994), considering data from Europe, Asia, Australia, New Zealand, and North America, underscored the increased risk of depression for patients with chronic medical illnesses. They concurred that most HIV-positive depressed patients have experienced an episode of depression before seroconverting. They speculated that American studies included larger percentages of medically healthy subjects, diminishing the rates of mood disorders that would be detected in a medically compromised HIV-positive sample.

Psychiatric inpatients, a group at much higher risk for depression than the general population, are also at increased risk for HIV (Cournos et al. 1991). Sacks et al. (1992) found that 25 of 350 (7%) acutely ill psychiatric inpatients tested seropositive for HIV. Mahler et al. (1994), testing blood samples from alcoholic inpatients, found that rates of HIV (10.4%) were even higher than in the general psychiatric inpatient population. For many reasons, psychiatric patients may represent an especially vulnerable group.

Although HIV itself produces subtle neuropsychological changes in humans, depression is an entity distinct from primary HIV infection. Stern et al. (1991) found no evidence of depression in homosexual male subjects with early cognitive dysfunction presumed secondary to HIV. Perkins et al. (1995) found that complaints of fatigue and insomnia in HIV-positive homosexual men were associated with dysphoric mood and other depressive symptoms rather than with HIV disease progression. Perry and Fishman (1993) similarly found no association between depression and HIV disease progression or immune status.

If depression is not a usual central nervous system manifestation of HIV, what about the medications used to treat HIV and its attendant opportunistic infections? HIV-positive individuals typically follow a regimen of multiple prescriptions including antiretrovirals (e.g., zidovudine and stavudine), protease inhibitors (e.g., ritonavir and indinavir), antivirals (e.g., acyclovir and foscarnet), antibiotics (e.g., trimethoprim/sulfamethoxazole and dapsone), and others. The relationship between depression and this polypharmacy is probably complex and multifactorial. For instance, in addition to the chemical effects of medication, pills may have psychological meaning to the patient such as "patient-hood" or a state of increased vulnerability and dependence. Yet, to our knowledge, no well-controlled studies exist documenting the relationship between mood and HIV medications. With the exception of the relatively new protease inhibitors, these medications have been used extensively in clinical settings. Clinical impressions and the paucity of case reports suggest that depression is probably a rare side effect of these treatments.

In part because of the development of protease inhibitors that can reduce viral loads to nondetectable levels and in part because of improved PCP prophylaxis regimens, AIDS has been transformed from an acutely lethal disease to a chronic illness marked by a reasonable potential for long-term survival. The evolution of the AIDS era has also been characterized by a shift in social sentiment, thanks in part to projects like the AIDS Quilt and to the increased visibility of HIV-positive celebrities including Rock Hudson, Magic Johnson, and Arthur Ashe. Improved prognosis and decreased social stigma contribute to making HIV less "depressing." Nonetheless, it is still a significant and potentially deadly stressor affecting a mostly young and previously vigorous segment of our population.

Despite an intuition to the contrary, depression does not appear to be inevitable in the face of HIV infection. The great majority of HIV-positive individuals are *not* depressed. Prior history of depression, current substance abuse, and greater degree of medical disability may predispose subgroups to depression but not necessarily to a greater degree than an HIV-negative or other medically ill cohort. Because both clinicians and patients may be inclined erroneously to attribute fatigue, insomnia, decreased libido, and weight loss to primary HIV infection or medication side effects, it is important to remember that an individual with these complaints should be evaluated for a mood disorder. Although depression is not the inevitable outcome of HIV, when its symptoms are present, the patient should be treated appropriately.

Treating Depression

Depression is a syndrome associated with considerable morbidity and dysfunction (Judd et al. 1996; Wells et al. 1989). For an individual coping with the already considerable pressures of HIV, depression is an additional—but, fortunately, eminently treatable—burden. The treatment of depression in any population requires the clinician to select among a large array of pharmacological and nonpharmacological alternatives. Although it is beyond the scope of this chapter to discuss the considerable range of somatic options available to the psychiatrist, suffice it to say that the usual treatments (e.g., selective serotonin reuptake inhibitors, tricyclic antidepressants, and electroconvulsive therapy) appear effective in (mostly open) trials with HIV-positive depressed subjects (Markowitz et al. 1994; Rabkin and Rabkin 1994). The presence of comorbid HIV infection should not confuse the clinician: depression is still depression, and the usual rules apply with only slight modification.

Nonpharmacological alternatives for treating depression have considerable appeal in an HIV-positive population. For individuals bound to the polypharmacy of current anti-HIV regimens, the mere thought of an additional pill may seem intolerable. For the clinician, complicated drug-drug interactions may make nonpharmacological choices preferable. For HIV-positive women, most of whom are in their childbearing years, the teratogenic risks of pharmacotherapy may complicate already difficult decisions about childbearing (Swartz et al. 1997). Some individuals may desire psychotherapy in addition to antidepressant medication to help them more effectively manage life stressors and diminish precipitants of the depression.

Psychotherapy is thus an appealing treatment option. In addition to avoiding the problems associated with pharmacotherapy, antidepressant psychotherapy offers the patient a way to both treat the depression and explore salient issues. HIV infection is an important life event with significant psychological consequences, and patients may want or need an opportunity to address them. Although each individual processes the challenges of HIV differently, some experiences are common to the HIV-positive population (Adler and Beckett 1989). For instance, within the gay community, HIV-infected individuals typically face the loss of lovers, groups of friends, and entire networks in addition to their own illness. Intravenous drug users, confronted with evidence of their infection and failing physical health, may vacillate between a renewed struggle to overcome their addiction and an impulse to give up hope. Infected women grapple with questions of childbearing, child care, and potentially infected offspring. All will confront their mortality, experience an interruption of their expected life trajectory, struggle with social stigma, and come into close and frequent contact with the medical establishment. A psychotherapy structured to address these issues offers clear advantages to HIV-positive patients.

Psychotherapy and HIV

Descriptions of psychotherapeutic approaches to HIV-positive patients derived from clinical experience are common in the literature (see Adler and Beckett 1989 and O'Connor 1997). Reports of psychotherapies tailored to treat depression in this population are less common (see Markowitz et al. 1993 and Targ et al. 1994), and randomized treatment trials are rare. Kelly et al. (1993) randomly assigned 68 depressed HIV-positive men to eight sessions of either cognitive-behavioral group therapy, a social support group, or a no-treatment control condition. They found that both active interventions produced a decrease in depressive symptoms. Targ et al. (1994) randomized 20 mildly to moderately depressed HIV-positive men to 12 sessions of a skills training group therapy with or without fluoxetine (20 mg/day). Both groups experienced a reduction of depressive symptoms, and there were no significant differences between the medicated and unmedicated groups.

Markowitz et al. (1995) published the only comparative study of individual psychotherapies for HIV-positive patients. Thirty-two depressed HIV-positive subjects (mostly men) were randomized to 16 weeks of either IPT or supportive psychotherapy (SP). IPT, a manualized individual psychotherapy specifically designed for the treatment of depression, produced better results in this population than a nonspecific supportive psychotherapy, although both groups improved. IPT not only lowered Hamilton Rating Scale for Depression (Hamilton 1960) scores but also led to dramatic changes in relationships, careers, and life goals. These data represent preliminary findings from a now complete larger study ($N = 101$) comparing IPT, CBT, SP, and imipramine plus SP (Markowitz et al., in press). In the completed study, subjects were mostly male (85%), gay or bisexual (80%), and white (58%). Although all groups improved, subjects who received IPT alone or imipramine plus SP had significantly greater improvement in depressive symptoms than those receiving CBT or SP alone (see Figure 5–1). The authors speculate that some of the properties of IPT such as encouragement to make life changes and recognition of the connection between mood and real-life events may be inherently more helpful to HIV-positive patients with depressive symptoms—who face a surfeit of such life events—than the cognitive restructuring and refocusing tech-

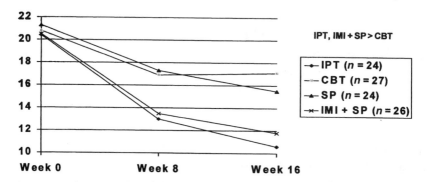

Figure 5–1. Hamilton Rating Scale for Depression score for intent-to-treat sample ($N = 101$). IPT, interpersonal psychotherapy; IMI, imipramine; SP, supportive psychotherapy; CBT, cognitive-behavioral therapy.

niques employed in CBT. These aspects of IPT are more fully elaborated later in this chapter. Limitations of the preceding studies include constricted patient demographics (i.e., primarily homosexual, relatively well-educated men, not all of whom met strict DSM criteria for a current mood disorder), small numbers of subjects per cell, and the absence of comparisons of group psychotherapy with individual psychotherapy.

Although the data are limited, IPT is the only psychotherapeutic modality to demonstrate a statistically significant and clinically meaningful advantage over other psychotherapies in the treatment of depressed, HIV-positive subjects. Until other approaches are codified, tested, and shown to have efficacy with this population, current information suggests that IPT is the scientifically proven nonpharmacological treatment of choice for HIV-positive individuals with depressive symptoms.

IPT for Depressed HIV-Positive Individuals

IPT was developed by the late Gerald L. Klerman and Myrna M. Weissman for the treatment of moderately severe outpatient depression (Klerman et al. 1984) and modified by Markowitz, Klerman, and the late Samuel Perry for the treatment of depression in a depressed HIV-positive population (IPT-HIV) (Markowitz et al. 1993). IPT (and IPT-HIV) is a time-limited, focused psychotherapy that emphasizes the connection between mood and life events. Because seroconversion produces a cascade of life events (e.g., doctors' appointments, conflict with sexual partners, fears of inadvertent disclosure, and often career changes), a model that pays particular attention to these changes meshes with the immediate concerns of HIV-positive patients.

Time Limit

IPT is administered for a predetermined, limited number of sessions (typically 12–16 weekly sessions). As Markowitz et al. (1993) reported, early concerns that a brief therapy might be inadequate for patients facing a terminal illness were allayed by patients' internal sense that time was precious. HIV-positive individuals, facing shortened futures, often want to make rapid, substantial changes in their lives. IPT therapists predict improvement in a few months' time and encourage patients to enact hitherto unfulfilled dreams. The therapy's time limitation fits easily and sensibly with the HIV-positive individual's time-sensitive agenda. Time is of the essence in the lives of our patients and in an era of a severely taxed mental health care system. IPT's structure naturally addresses these demands.

Here-and-Now Treatment

IPT maintains a focus on the here and now, or current life events. Depressed patients may be inclined to ruminate about prior disappointing relationships, dwelling on the past without making progress in the present. The IPT therapist helps the patient to focus on a current interpersonal problem area and encourages changes in the moment. HIV-positive patients may drift to either the past or the future, longing for their preinfection lifestyles and friends or prematurely dwelling on anticipated suffering and death. Although the therapist attends to these concerns (i.e., helps the patient to mourn prior losses or address particular fears about the future), the here-and-now focus of IPT requires that the patient examine current life issues. With HIV-positive patients, this approach can be particularly helpful: although the future may be uncertain, a fulfilling and happy present life is often possible. IPT facilitates this hopeful, practical outlook.

Patient-Therapist Relationship

The therapist treating an HIV-positive patient can be threatened by intense countertransferential feelings including irrational fears of contamination, fears of death and disease, and perhaps shame, disgust, or excitement about unfamiliar sexual practices (Cadwell 1997). By helping the patient see that options exist when he or she believed there were none, the IPT therapist establishes a positive, optimistic stance that counteracts the patient's depressed attitudes. The therapist, who is required to have some familiarity with HIV and its treatments in order to help the patient gain expertise, can help demystify the illness and correct misinformation acquired by the patient or his or her family members. In addition, IPT provides a hopeful, optimistic, and pragmatic framework for the therapist. The IPT structure helps the therapist avoid burnout and regulate potentially interfering countertransference. In other words, IPT provides the therapist with a system to help manage potentially overwhelming clinical material.

By contrast, the patient may bring to the therapeutic situation a long-standing mistrust of caregivers. Gays, ethnic minority groups, substance abusers, and women have long histories of mistreatment by the psychiatric establishment (Lerman 1996). The therapist should elicit a history of prior psychotherapeutic experiences and work hard to establish a therapeutic alliance. By communicating a willingness to suspend moral judgment and to explore all aspects of the patient's life, the therapist can help establish a basis of trust in the therapeutic relationship. The therapist's expertise in and familiarity with HIV can also be helpful in allaying patients' suspicions about the medical establishment. Without offering unrealistic promises about the course of disease progression, the therapist can provide the patient with current, reliable information about the nature of depression and HIV. A relaxed, conversational approach and the supportive stance of the IPT therapist may also help relieve patient discomfort with therapy. If the patient becomes too medically ill to travel to sessions, the therapist can further consolidate the relationship by visiting the patient in the hospital and conducting sessions by phone as needed.

Sick Role and Diagnosis

During the initial phase of IPT, the therapist conducts a careful diagnostic interview including a thorough medical history. This information enables the therapist to formally diagnose the patient as having a depressive episode. By labeling the disorder, the therapist objectifies the patient's symptoms and renders them ego dystonic. Whereas the patient had previously felt "bad" or "flawed," a formal diagnosis legitimizes the patient's illness. The therapist gives the patient the sick role (Parsons 1951) and instills the notion that he or she has a treatable illness. The sick role relieves the patient of some social obligations while assigning him or her the responsibility of working to get better. For IPT, the job description includes attending sessions, discussing relevant material during sessions, and working on interpersonal problems between sessions.

For HIV-positive patients, the therapist diagnoses two disorders, depression and HIV. The sick role description associated with HIV includes seeking appropriate medical care, negotiating with the often complex medical insurance system, and becoming knowledgeable and educated about HIV. When appropriate, the therapist can point out the ways in which the patient is *not* ill, underscoring the fact that the asymptomatic period of the infection can persist for years and that medications such as the protease inhibitors may improve prognosis.

Psychoeducation

IPT traditionally incorporates significant psychoeducation about depression. The patient is encouraged to identify symptoms, understand the relationship between mood and life events, and learn about pathophysiology and treatments. In addition to becoming experts about depression, HIV-positive patients are encouraged to become experts about HIV. Many patients enter IPT with misconceptions and lack of information about the nature and course of HIV illness and about advances in its treatment. The patient may be unaware of the existence of nonprogressors, the potential for long asymptomatic periods, or the availability of new medical treatments such as viral load testing and protease inhibitors. The IPT therapist should impart information, correct misinformation, and encourage the patient to develop resources outside of therapy.

IPT Problem Areas

IPT-HIV retains the four traditional IPT problem areas: grief, role disputes, role transitions, and interpersonal deficits (Klerman et al. 1984). These categories lend themselves well to the issues confronting an HIV-positive patient population, and no specific modifications have been necessary. Given the surfeit of life events experienced by the HIV-positive patient, the first three categories usually suffice. Contracting HIV is a transforming event—a role transition by definition—essentially obviating the need for the interpersonal deficits category. Descriptions and examples of each problem area follow.

Grief

In IPT, grief refers to complicated bereavement. In other words, someone has died, and the patient experiences a depressive reaction that exceeds the scope of normal grieving. Some individuals experience an inability to grieve, whereas others experience a protracted, exaggerated grief reaction. In the environments of HIV-positive individuals, death is an unfortunately common occurrence. The communities most directly affected by the epidemic have witnessed the demise of huge segments of the population. The sheer numbers of deaths can numb an appropriate mourning response. Grief for lost loved ones or close acquaintances can become confused with premature grief for the patient's anticipated death, with some depressed HIV-positive patients feeling and behaving as if life were over from the moment they seroconverted. At other times, the loss of a particular individual is amplified by the multiple antecedent losses experienced by the patient, confounding the mourning process.

The therapist seeks to identify for the patient a particular loss or losses associated with the onset of depressive symptoms. He or she encourages the patient to appropriately mourn the deceased individual by helping the patient reconstruct the relationship, acknowledging both the positive and negative aspects of the connection. It is important to acknowledge multiple losses, if they have occurred, while focusing the patient's attention on the most affectively meaningful material. Concretely, the therapist encourages the patient to look at photos, review the memories of the death and funeral, visit grave sites, go through personal effects, and so forth to facilitate the mourning process. As this process progresses, the therapist also encourages appropriate substitutions for the lost relationship.

Case Example

Mr. B is a 47-year-old gay white male whose insomnia, weight loss, and anergia began immediately after the precipitous death of his lover 2 years before from a boating accident. Formerly an active member of the community, Mr. B withdrew from many of his friends after the funeral. Mr. B and his lover, who had both been diagnosed HIV-positive 6 months before the accident, responded to the news by agreeing to share responsibilities for the household, health care, and caretaking. Together they enrolled in HIV educational seminars and planned to participate in phase III trials of (at that time, otherwise unavailable) protease inhibitors. They were both asymptomatic at the time of diagnosis and anticipated an extended period of shared health.

As therapy began, it became clear that, although greatly saddened by his lover's death, Mr. B was also enraged. He had expected to face a future with HIV in good company and experienced the death as an abandonment. Mr. B's depression seemed related to these unresolved feelings, and his treatment focus was formulated as complicated bereavement. His therapist encouraged Mr. B to verbalize his negative and positive feelings about his deceased lover. They discussed in detail his lover's refusal to wear a life preserver on the night of the accident and Mr. B's belief that this refusal contributed to his lover's drowning. As Mr. B expressed his sadness, rage, and fears about the future, his symptoms receded. Mr. B was encouraged to reach out to old friends and seek other sources of support. As treatment ended, Mr. B found himself able to share both future uncertainties and current pleasures with old friends.

Role Dispute

A role dispute refers to a relationship in difficulty because of nonreciprocal expectations of two parties. In some cases the conflict is obvious and overt; in others it is insidious or covert. Treating a role dispute has been described as unilateral couples therapy (Markowitz 1997). The therapist's goal is to identify the dispute for the patient and connect the dispute to the onset and maintenance of depression. Once the dispute is clarified, the therapist helps the patient to identify options in the relationship and encourages the patient to enact changes. A satisfactory resolution would include either improvement in the relationship or, when appropriate, its dissolution.

The diagnosis of HIV introduces an important and potentially problematic element into all significant relationships. Conflict may erupt when an HIV-negative partner refuses physical contact with an HIV-positive former lover or when a "closeted" HIV-positive homosexual reveals his serostatus, and de facto his sexual preferences, to his uninformed parents. Disputes may emerge in the workplace when an employee develops HIV-related special needs and an employer is unsympathetic or when fears of discrimination prevent an employee from revealing his or her status. Role disputes are often relevant treatment foci for this population.

As the case of Ms. C illustrates, revealing (or not revealing) serostatus to a sexual partner adds a new, lethal dimension to the disputes fostered by all sexually transmitted diseases. Like syphilis in the past, the sexual transgressions of a partner can lead to serious infection in the nontransgressor, creating irreconcilable differences between partners.

Case Example

Ms. C, a 27-year-old single Hispanic female, learned that she was HIV-positive during routine prenatal care for an unplanned pregnancy. Six months after electively terminating the pregnancy, she began developing depressive symptoms including hypersomnia, weight gain, anergia, and passive suicidal ideation. When she entered therapy Ms. C was preoccupied with how she became infected with HIV. Although she had been promiscuous in high school, she had no other risk factors. She had been in a monogamous relationship over the past year with her boyfriend, and he denied being HIV-positive. However, she thought he had begun to act "a little funny" after she was diagnosed. Initially she attributed his distress to her decision to abort the pregnancy but later began to wonder if he had lied to her. She noted that he would disappear for hours at a time and that he was willing to engage in unprotected intercourse with her, despite his alleged negative serostatus. He had a history of drug and alcohol use, but she believed him to be in remission.

Therapy focused on making explicit the dispute between Ms. C and her boyfriend. Ms. C was encouraged to verbalize her suspicions first in therapy and later with her boyfriend. Initially reluctant to confront him, Ms. C finally admitted that she did not think that he had ever been tested and that he actively avoided medical doctors. Ms. C felt that she could voice concerns that he had never been tested but was unable to state her increasingly strong belief that he had infected her. The boyfriend denied that he had never been tested but finally agreed to "repeat" testing. Not surprisingly, his antibody titers were positive. After the boyfriend's formal diagnosis, the couple began fighting constantly about household finances and responsibilities.

After using communication analysis to understand and make explicit the subtext of the arguments and role-play to prepare Ms. C to confront her boyfriend, Ms. C finally accused her boyfriend of infecting her. The boyfriend stormed out of the apartment in response but did not deny the accusations. Ms. C felt that she "got [her] answer" and left the relationship to live, on an interim basis, with her mother. Although sad about the departure of her ex-boyfriend, Ms. C felt satisfied that she had been able to express her anger directly.

As treatment ended, Ms. C remained dysphoric in the face of the recent dissolution of her relationship, but her suicidal ideation and neurovegetative symptoms had receded. She felt relieved to have left a relationship that she considered dishonest and planned to join a support group for HIV-positive women.

Role Transition

A role transition is defined as any major life event or change in social roles. Examples include starting a new job, moving to a new city, becoming a parent, divorcing, marrying, graduating, being promoted, being fired, joining the army, and so forth. The category of role transitions includes losses such as suffering a household fire, financial setbacks, or physical infirmity. (In IPT, grief refers specifically to the death of a *person*.) Treatment includes identifying the transition, linking it to the onset of the mood disorder, and helping the patient to reevaluate both the old and new roles. Patients, particularly once depressed, often idealize the old role and devalue the new one; in IPT they learn to see the positive and negative aspects of both roles with the help of an objective yet optimistic therapist. When treating HIV-positive patients, the therapist and patient strive to find the silver lining of HIV infection (Markowitz et al. 1995) as the central task in making a successful role transition. The time pressure induced by HIV infection can make time seem more valuable, leading the patient to reassess his or her life priorities. The silver lining may come in the form of a newfound freedom to actively pursue previously deferred life goals or the unexpected impetus to strengthen previously neglected significant relationships.

HIV diagnosis carries with it an inherent role transition. Even if the outcome has been anticipated or expected, testing positive changes your life and your perspective on life. An otherwise healthy individual is suddenly confronted with a terminal illness that carries with it fears of contagion and suffering; an endless array of doctors, blood tests, and medications; and a tremendous uncertainty about course and outcome. Unlike many other life-threatening illnesses, HIV also brings with it significant social stigma. In addition to facing the challenges of the illness itself, HIV-positive patients can anticipate confronting the prejudices of insurance carriers, employers, and entire segments of the population. It introduces a complex element into all intimate relationships, whether or not the partner is also HIV-positive. HIV brings the patient head to head with a medical establishment that is itself uncertain about the best course of treatment and is unable to predict outcomes.

Beyond testing positive, HIV-positive patients go through multiple additional transitions as the disease progresses. The diagnosis of an AIDS-defining illness, a significant drop in T cells, or a rise in viral load titers often represent important transitions for patients. As medical treatments have become more effective, full recovery after a single opportunistic infection is the norm. Yet some patients, having experienced one infection, believe that the specter of death is fast approaching and may become very demoralized or depressed. In the era of protease inhibitors, some may feel entitled to an indefinite disease-free period and become depressed in the face of an unexpected, and to them untenable, setback. At some point, patients will mourn the loss of their former, uninfected selves and participate in anticipatory mourning for expected suffering and death. These issues are also handled as role transitions in IPT.

For a drug-using population, testing positive for an AIDS-defining illness may coincide with a transition to sobriety or abstinence. In addition to managing the demands of HIV, a patient in newly achieved remission from a drug or alcohol addiction struggles with the urge to "pick up" and the loss of pleasure from previously enjoyable—if maladaptive—behaviors. This situation represents an additional role transition that can be addressed in IPT. In this case, the therapist's challenge is to suspend moral judgment and help the patient mourn the loss of the pleasurable aspects of the old role while reinforcing the beneficial and pleasurable aspects of abstinence. Dealing with HIV and abstinence may be called a double transition; the patient's success in coping with abstinence may be used to bolster his or her handling of HIV infection, or vice versa.

Because of the nature of this illness, all HIV-positive patients can be identified as experiencing a role transition. Whether this transition is central to the depression and hence the IPT treatment requires the clinical judgment of the therapist. For some patients, IPT focuses on two problem areas (e.g., grief and role transition).

Case Example

Dr. D is a 35-year-old single white male physician whose lover had died during their medical residencies 8 years ago. Dr. D had been diagnosed as HIV-positive at the time of his lover's death but had been relatively healthy and able to function as a physician until age 33. At that age, Dr. D developed a debilitating peripheral neuropathy that caused him to miss many days of work. Nevertheless, he continued to function as an internist on a reduced schedule. With great hope, he had enrolled in a protease inhibitor trial and was intensely disappointed when, instead of improving, his health declined. Dr. D developed severe insomnia, anorexia, and dysphoria after requiring a brief hospitalization for the treatment of cytomegalovirus (CMV) retinitis.

Dr. D was diagnosed with major depression, and his IPT problem area was conceptualized as a role transition. It became apparent in treatment that Dr. D had handled the role of being HIV-positive very well until his health began to decline. Deprived of the capacity to work regularly, Dr. D felt that "life [had] no meaning." He was also frightened by the bout of CMV retinitis because a similar episode had heralded the demise of his deceased lover. Dr. D focused on how he had turned to his work after his lover's death to find meaning and pleasure in his life. He admitted that he had neglected all other aspects of his life in the process, so that without his work, his life was in fact relatively impoverished. The silver lining of Dr. D's illness was the opportunity to rediscover areas of life that he had ignored after medical school. The therapist encouraged Dr. D to live out his fantasy of residing in the country. Dr. D made plans to move temporarily back to his parents' farm, where he would have the opportunity to walk and garden, pastimes he had enjoyed in adolescence. He also admitted that his parents could provide him with some much-needed physical and emotional assistance, a support he lacked in his urban apartment miles from his family.

Therapy also focused on Dr. D's sadness about the deterioration of his health and vivid memories of his lover's terrible final months. Finding relief in the opportunity to share and explore his fears, Dr. D admitted that treatments had improved greatly in the 8 years since his lover's death. Although he continued to express disappointment about the failure of the protease inhibitor to provide a "cure," he acknowledged that he could reasonably expect a period of relative health and tranquility in the country. As treatment concluded, Dr. D showed no evidence of depression, and he looked forward to his move. In his last session, Dr. D confided that he hoped to work part-time at a small clinic near his parents' farm if he remained well but felt relieved to be excused from the demands of a full-time clinical practice.

Interpersonal Deficits

Interpersonal deficits is a category reserved for patients with a long-standing history of impoverished interpersonal relationships, including some patients who would meet criteria for avoidant or narcissistic personality disorders. These patients lack life events, the fulcrum around which IPT works, and therefore patients in this category generally have poorer outcomes than other IPT patients. Because HIV generates life events, you can essentially *always* select one of the other three categories. The life-altering effects of HIV may paradoxically contribute to IPT's success with this population.

The case of Dr. D described earlier might have been appropriate for the interpersonal deficits category because he led a very isolated, bereft existence with little human contact outside of his work. Because we preferentially selected one of the other three problem areas and because the depression was clearly related to his deteriorating health, a role transition proved a much more fruitful arena for exploration. (Alternately, Dr. D's case could have focused on reawakened unresolved grief over his lover's death in response to developing CMV retinitis.)

Special Issues

Psychotherapy and HIV-Positive Women

The few extant controlled treatment studies (discussed earlier) enrolled primarily male subjects, characteristically omitting women from HIV-related treatment trials (Levine 1990). Neither Kelly et al. (1993) nor Targ et al. (1994) included *any* women in their analyses. Only 15% of the 101 subjects enrolled by Markowitz et al. (in press) were women. There are no published data documenting the efficacy of psychotherapy for depressed HIV-positive women, although the potential teratogenicity of pharmacotherapy makes psychotherapy a particularly appealing option for these women of (mostly) childbearing age.

Our unpublished analysis of 23 women treated with 16 weeks

of either IPT, CBT, or SP demonstrated that depressive symptoms diminished, regardless of treatment condition (H. A. Swartz, J. C. Markowitz, L. A. Spielman, unpublished data, January 1997). Our sample included nine women enrolled in the Markowitz et al. (in press) study. In both completer ($n = 11$) and intent-to-treat ($n = 23$) analyses, Beck Depression Inventory (Beck 1978) scores showed a statistically significant decrease from intake to termination. Hamilton Rating Scale for Depression scores showed a statistically significant drop in completer analyses and approached statistical significance in intent-to-treat analyses. Perhaps because of the small sample size, there were no statistically significant differences among treatment conditions. The high level of attrition (50%) is typical of our experience with this population and poses one of the greatest methodological challenges when conducting research with this group. We have reported elsewhere the case of an HIV-positive pregnant women whose mood and interpersonal relationships improved remarkably with 12 sessions of IPT (Swartz et al. 1997).

Compared with HIV-positive men, HIV-positive women are more likely to be poor, socioeconomically disadvantaged, and members of an ethnic minority group (Cambell 1990). HIV-positive women are generally less well educated than their male counterparts and are often single mothers responsible for both themselves and their (several, often HIV-positive) children. Unlike many gay men (the largest segment of the HIV-positive male population), HIV-positive women may get little support from established community organizations such as the Gay Men's Health Crisis or Body Positive. HIV-positive women may not even consider HIV infection their most pressing concern. Living in the inner city, they routinely endure stressors such as domestic violence, violent crime, inadequate housing, and single parenthood, unlike most HIV-positive men. Ward (1993, p. 413) quoted a poor, black, HIV-positive mother as saying, "You think AIDS is a problem? No way. I got real problems."

Our experience with this population suggests that, although they are difficult to engage in treatment (perhaps because of the numerous problems facing them), they benefit tremendously from the intervention once engaged. Given the difficult HIV-related decisions they face including disclosure to children (Lipson 1993), permanency planning, and childbearing (Goggin and Rabkin 1997), a treatment that incorporates some of the HIV-specific strategies outlined previously would probably suit the needs of this largely neglected population.

Protease Inhibitors

With the advent of the protease inhibitors and viral load testing, we have moved into a new phase of the epidemic. Today's expectations are that seropositive people will remain asymptomatic and live for longer periods. If not a cure, these treatments represent an important breakthrough for patients haunted by the protean assaults of this virus. For many individuals, these treatments bring hope and clinical improvement. But when the so-called magic eludes others who are ineligible for or fail treatment, the loss of hope can be devastating (e.g., the case of Dr. D described earlier). For those who "need to know," a treatment that prolongs life but offers no cure may mean years of added uncertainty, paradoxically encouraging patients to put their lives on hold. Some individuals, expecting to die imminently, had spent their savings, settled for suboptimal relationships, or divested themselves of their possessions. With successful protease inhibitor treatment, they are now faced with the long-term consequences of these short-term decisions.

We have yet to evaluate the effect of protease inhibitors on psychotherapy outcomes. IPT has been called a therapy of change, and it may be paradoxically more difficult to motivate an HIV-positive patient who is doing relatively well while taking protease inhibitors. The lethality of HIV acts as an agent of change, and less danger may mean less willingness to take psychotherapeutic and real-life risks. Lulled into the lassitude of the relatively well, patients may be less willing than their time-pressured counterparts to enact the dramatic changes that have been so gratifying for both our patients and those of us privileged to work with this population. On the other hand, some individuals shocked into action by their HIV diagnosis may have their resolve for self-improvement enhanced by the second chance provided by protease inhibitors.

As medical treatments continue to improve, the hopelessness that has been so integral to this epidemic may recede. Because IPT has been so effective in engendering hope when there was none, it may be reasonable to apply these principles to other medical conditions, such as pancreatic or lung cancer, where hopelessness still abounds.

IPT and Other Medically Ill Patients

Treating depression comorbid with HIV may inform the treatment of depression comorbid with other medical illnesses. Although the sociology and social stigma of HIV are unique, the principles of IPT for HIV can probably be generalized to other chronic, life-threatening medical conditions such as cancer, diabetes, and heart disease. Schulberg and colleagues (1996) treated depressed primary care patients in a medical setting with either nortriptyline ($n = 91$), IPT ($n = 93$), or a physician's usual care ($n = 92$). Patients receiving the specialized antidepressant treatment (either medication or IPT) showed greater, more rapid improvement, demonstrating that IPT has utility in a general medical setting. Schulberg and co-workers (1993) focus on adapting to limitations caused by physical morbidity as an example of an interpersonal role transition.

Maintenance Treatment

IPT is an acute treatment, and the changes depressed HIV-positive patients make in an acute 16-week time period are often dramatic. The question lingers, however, whether a maintenance phase is indicated after treatment remission. Maintenance treatment studies of HIV-negative patients with recurrent major depression suggest that relapse rates are high in the absence of ongoing active treatment (Frank et al. 1990). Because many HIV-positive patients have had prior episodes of depression (Markowitz et al. 1994), they may be at higher risk for relapse and therefore benefit from maintenance treatment, perhaps at a less frequent rate of sessions (e.g., monthly [Frank et al. 1990]). For individuals with single episodes, acute treatment may be sufficient.

Conclusion

IPT for the treatment of depressed HIV-positive men and women retains the basic principles of IPT but also includes important modifications to address the special needs of this population:

1. IPT-HIV addresses two medical illnesses—depression and HIV—requiring expertise of the therapist and education of the patient in both areas.
2. The multiple life events generated by HIV can be conceptualized as grief, a role transition, or a role dispute, obviating the need for the deficits category.
3. Grief work includes mourning the multiple deaths endured by this community and anticipatory mourning for the patient's own death.
4. Developing a therapeutic alliance with this often disenfranchised population requires special attention. The therapist maintains an open, friendly, nonjudgmental stance, especially around issues such as drug use and sexual practices that may have previously caused the patient to suffer from social stigma.
5. The therapist may act as a liaison to the patient's medical doctor, helping to interpret the often confusing and uncertain information offered about prognosis and treatment.
6. If patients become medically ill during the course of treatment, requiring hospitalization or becoming homebound, therapists are encouraged to visit patients, continuing therapy in the hospital or by phone as needed.
7. HIV-positive women may require additional modifications of IPT-HIV such as increased scheduling flexibility and liberal use of phone sessions.

Depression and HIV are both chronic but remitting and potentially suppressible illnesses. IPT may be the nonpharmacological treatment of choice for individuals experiencing these medical disorders simultaneously. IPT offers the HIV-positive patient and the therapist a systematic, interpersonally focused means of addressing both psychosocial stressors and depressive symptoms. Changes made in therapy are both rewarding for the patient and gratifying for the therapist. IPT offers hope to both patients and therapists in the face of two debilitating illnesses, HIV and depression.

References

Adler G, Beckett A: Psychotherapy of the patient with an HIV infection: some ethical and therapeutic dilemmas. Psychosomatics 30:203–208, 1989

Atkinson J, Grant I, Kennedy C, et al: Prevalence of psychiatric disorders among men infected with human immunodeficiency virus. Arch Gen Psychiatry 45:859–864, 1988

Cadwell SA: Transference and countertransference, in Treating the Psychological Consequences of HIV. Edited by O'Connor MF. San Francisco, CA, Jossey-Bass, 1997, pp 1–32

Cambell CA: Women and AIDS. Soc Sci Med 30:407–415, 1990

Cournos F, Empfield M, Horwath E, et al: HIV seroprevalence among patients admitted to two psychiatric hospitals. Am J Psychiatry 148:1225–1230, 1991

Frank E, Kupfer DJ, Perel JM, et al: Three year outcomes for maintenance therapies in recurrent depression. Arch Gen Psychiatry 47:1093–1099, 1990

Goggin KJ, Rabkin JG: Treating HIV-positive women, in Treating the Psychological Consequences of HIV. Edited by O'Connor MF. San Francisco, CA, Jossey-Bass, 1997, pp 195–223

Hamilton M: A rating scale for depression. J Neurol Neurosurg Psychiatry 23:56–62, 1960

Judd FK, Mijch AM: Depression in patients with HIV and AIDS. Aust N Z J Psychiatry 28:642–650, 1994

Judd LL, Paulus MP, Wells KB, et al: Socioeconomic burden of subsyndromal depressive symptoms and major depression in a sample of the general population. Am J Psychiatry 153:1411–1417, 1996

Kelly JA, Murphy DA, Bahr GR, et al: Outcome of cognitive-behavioral and support group brief therapies for depressed, HIV-infected persons. Am J Psychiatry 150:1679–1686, 1993

Klerman GL, Weissman MM, Rounsaville BJ, et al: Interpersonal Psychotherapy of Depression. New York, Basic Books, 1984

Lambert MJ, Bergin AE: The effectiveness of psychotherapy, in Handbook of Psychotherapy and Behavior Change, 4th Edition. Edited by Bergin AE, Garfield SL. New York, Wiley, 1994

Lerman H: Pigeonholing Women's Misery: A History and Critical Analysis of the Psychodiagnosis of Women in the Twentieth Century. New York, Basic Books, 1996

Levine C: Women and HIV/AIDS research: the barriers to equity. Evaluation Review 14:447–463, 1990

Lipsitz JD, William JBW, Rabkin JG, et al: Psychopathology in male and female intravenous drug users with and without HIV infection. Am J Psychiatry 151:1662–1668, 1994

Lipson M: What do you say to a child with AIDS? Hastings Cent Rep 23:6–12, 1993

Mahler J, Stebinger A, Yi D, et al: Reliability of admission history in predicting HIV infection among alcoholic inpatients. American Journal on Addictions 3:222–226, 1994

Markowitz JC: Interpersonal Psychotherapy for Dysthymic Disorder. Washington, DC, American Psychiatric Press, 1997

Markowitz JC, Klerman GL, Perry SW, et al: Interpersonal therapy for depressed HIV-seropositive patients, in New Applications of Interpersonal Therapy. Edited by Klerman GL, Weissman MM. Washington, DC, American Psychiatric Press, 1993, pp 199–224

Markowitz JC, Rabkin JG, Perry SW: Treating depression in HIV-positive patients. AIDS 8:403–412, 1994

Markowitz JC, Klerman GL, Clougherty KF, et al: Individual psychotherapies for depressed HIV-positive patients. Am J Psychiatry 152:1504–1509, 1995

Markowitz JC, Kocsis JH, Fishman B: Treatment of depressive symptoms in HIV-positive patients. Arch Gen Psychiatry (in press)

O'Connor MF (ed): Treating the Psychological Consequences of HIV. San Francisco, CA, Jossey-Bass, 1997

Parsons T: Illness and the role of the physician: a sociological perspective. Am J Orthopsychiatry 21:452–460, 1951

Perkins DO, Stern RA, Golden RN, et al: Mood disorders in HIV infection: prevalence and risk factors in a nonepicenter of the AIDS epidemic. Am J Psychiatry 151:233–263, 1994

Perkins DO, Leserman J, Stern RA, et al: Somatic symptoms and HIV infection: relationship to depressive symptoms and indicators of HIV disease. Am J Psychiatry 152:1776–1781, 1995

Perry S, Fishman B: Depression and HIV: how does one affect the other? JAMA 250:2609–2610, 1993

Rabkin JG, Rabkin R: Treatment of depression in HIV infection. Infections in Medicine 11:601–612, 1994

Rabkin JG, Rabkin R, Harrison W: Imipramine effects on mood and immune status in depressed patients with HIV illness: preliminary findings. Paper presented at Neurobehavioral Findings in AIDS Research conference. Washington, DC, September 1991

Sacks M, Dermatis H, Looser-Ott S, et al: Undetected HIV infection among acutely ill psychiatric inpatients. Am J Psychiatry 149:544–545, 1992

Schulberg HC, Scott CP, Madonia MJ, et al: Applications of interpersonal psychotherapy to depression in primary care practice, in New Applications of Interpersonal Therapy. Edited by Klerman GL, Weissman MM. Washington, DC, American Psychiatric Press, 1993, pp 265–291

Schulberg HC, Block MR, Madonia MJ, et al: Treating major depression in primary care practice. Arch Gen Psychiatry 53:913–919, 1996

Stern Y, Marder K, Bell K, et al: Multidisciplinary baseline assessment of homosexual men with and without human immunodeficiency virus III: neurologic and neuropsychological findings. Arch Gen Psychiatry 48:131–138, 1991

Swartz HA, Markowitz JC, Spinelli MG: Interpersonal psychotherapy of a depressed, pregnant, HIV-positive woman. Journal of Psychotherapy Practice and Research 6:166–178, 1997

Targ EF, Karasic DH, Diefenbach PN, et al: Structured group therapy and fluoxetine to treat depression in HIV-positive persons. Psychosomatics 35:132–137, 1994

Ward MC: A different disease: HIV/AIDS and health care for women in poverty. Cult Med Psychiatry 17:413–430, 1993

Weiner J: Is depression inevitable in the face of AIDS? AIDS Reader March/April:66–72, 1996

Wells KB, Stewart A, Hays RD, et al: The functioning and well-being of depressed patients: results from the medical outcomes study. JAMA 262:914–919, 1989

Afterword

John C. Markowitz, M.D.

The preceding chapters provide a glimpse into the state of interpersonal psychotherapy (IPT) on the eve of the twenty-first century. IPT has clearly come a great distance in the past 25 years and promises to go further. Other chapters might certainly have been included had space existed, including reviews of research testing IPT as a treatment for depressed geriatric patients, depressed primary care patients, dysthymic patients, and bipolar patients; preliminary research on patients with anxiety disorders; and so forth. The dissemination of IPT among clinicians, training, and certification issues also deserve attention and will affect the future of IPT (Markowitz 1997). A review 10 years hence will no doubt embrace a far greater range of IPT treatment studies and reveal far more about its clinical spread.

The utility of IPT is defined by the DSM-IV (American Psychiatric Association 1994) diagnoses for which it has been tested. It is important to conceive of IPT as one treatment choice among many. Considerable research will be required to develop differential therapeutics (Frances et al. 1984): that is, the appropriate selection of particular treatments, and their combinations, for particular patients with particular disorders. When IPT should be used alone, when in combination with pharmacotherapy, and when not at all remains to be definitively determined.

References

American Psychiatric Association: Diagnostic and Statistical Manual of Mental Disorders, 4th Edition. Washington, DC, American Psychiatric Association, 1994

Frances A, Clarkin JF, Perry S: Differential Therapeutics in Psychiatry: The Art and Science of Treatment Selection. New York, Brunner/ Mazel, 1984

Markowitz JC: The future of interpersonal psychotherapy. Journal of Psychotherapy Practice and Research 6:294–299, 1997

Index

Page numbers in **boldface** type indicate tables or figures.

Preventive treatment, for depression.
    See Maintenance interpersonal
    psychotherapy
Primary care, practice guidelines, 3
Primary care patients, IPT for, 12–13,
    19
Protease inhibitors, and IPT-HIV,
    150–151
Protective service agencies, and
    IPT-A, 56–57
Psychoeducation, in IPT-HIV,
    140–141
Psychotherapy. *See also* Interpersonal
    psychotherapy
    HIV and, 135–137
    HIV-positive women and,
        148–150

Research, on IPT-A
    controlled clinical trial, 61–62
    open clinical trial, 59–61
    therapist training, 59
Response, predictors of, for IPT
        treatment of mood disorders,
        7–9
Role disputes
    IPT for, 5
    IPT-A for, 45–46
    IPT-BN for, 113–114
    IPT-HIV for, 143–144
Role transitions
    IPT for, 5
    IPT-A for, 46–48
    IPT-BN for, 114
    IPT-HIV for, 144–147

School involvement, in IPT-A
    sessions, 40–41

School refusal, IPT-A for, 55–56
Sexual abuse, IPT-A for, 57
Sexual identity problems,
        adolescents with, IPT-A for, 58
Short-term focal psychotherapy.
    See Interpersonal
    psychotherapy
Sick role in
    IPT-A, 41–42
    IPT-HIV, 139–140
Single-parent families, adolescents
    in, IPT-A for, 49–51
Social phobia, IPT for, 16–18
Substance abuse
    IPT for, 15–16
    IPT-A for, 56
Subsyndromally depressed
        hospitalized elderly patients,
        IPC for, 21–22
Suicidal patients, IPT-A for, 54

Therapist training program, IPT-A
        research in, 59–62
Therapists, association with IPT-M
        outcomes, 86
Time factors
    for IPT-A sessions, 40
    limits for IPT-HIV sessions,
        137–138
Training, in IPT, 24–25. *See also*
        Therapist training program
Treatment contract, in IPT-A, 42
Treatment specificity, association
        with IPT-M outcomes
    psychobiological variables, 82–90
    psychological variables, 80–82